Tantric Sex Positions

The Complete Sex Guide to Forge a Deep Connection Through Sex Massage, Breathing, Intimacy and Techniques That Involve Your Whole Bodies and Live the Best Romantic Experience

JESSICA RYAN

Legal and disclaimer

Table of contents

Introduction

Tantra is the only spiritual path that sees the 360 ° relationship between men and women, and even if there are not many maps or disciplines that are valid in the culture of pleasure and eros at this time, it is very good to use tantric practices. It makes you feel good and grow without harming yourself or others.

The ancient technique of tantra teaches us to open all the knots that hinder the discovery of the possessions of our bodies and our love partners in a simple and gentle way. The biggest secret in these techniques is that desire and its fulfillment have no boundaries within us: we can grow together there, without one ever exhausting the other.

Tension, anxiety, physical and psychological fatigue disappear soon, in this discovery of a different sexuality, opening the way to tenderness, relaxation, first, and then to a dimension of knowledge that goes well beyond the physical relationship, up to joining the energies more subtle, the deep self of the two partners.

Based on authentic Indian and Tibetan texts and direct teachings from tantric masters, this book identifies the "western way" for tantra, the theoretical and practical way for deep life - through the energy of love - love, mutual curiosity, and excitement the senses. The word tantra has the right meaning: technology. It was born like the philosophy of tantric love, which uses special sexual techniques to bring abundance and intimacy into a relationship. Tantra - also known as sex yoga - is primarily love and a new way to see life.

Much is written and read about Tantra, but often these are overly learned books, dedicated to understanding one of the most complex and occult spiritual traditions, or trivially popular, aimed at interpreting Tantrism in a magical key.

This manual, on the other hand, represents a successful attempt to integrate into our culture some of the principles and above all the practices that Tantra dedicates to sexuality. The exercises, techniques and rituals he proposes, in fact, can be easily understood and performed by all of us, in everyday life.

In particular, through tantric teaching, the book helps: to become more aware of our body and its needs; to increase pleasure and to control sexual energy; to rediscover desire in all its intensity; to live eroticism as an exchange and sharing of love; to transform passion into affectionate attention.

Furthermore, this book describes the role of relationships, love and intimacy in modern Tantric traditions; teaches us to open our hearts - to ourselves and to others - through the exploration of our sexuality; he offers us tantric techniques for accessing spiritual experiences and reaching higher states of consciousness. Once these energies are released, we can make love for hours, or meditate in union with the partner to strengthen the couple's intimacy.

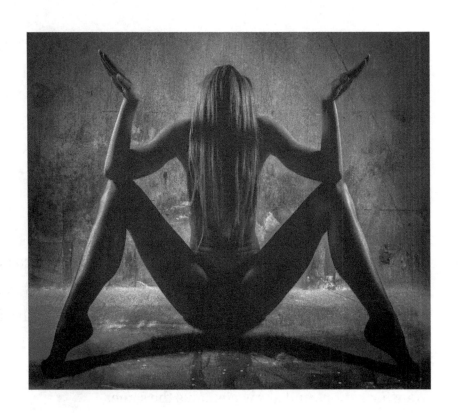

Chapter 1. Tantra history, myths and cultures

Tantrism is a holistic approach to life that examines the universe from an individual's perspective: the study of macrocosms through the study of microcosms. This is spiritual science, regardless of dogma or belief, based on experience, observation and practice.

It uses all the basic sciences, namely astrology, numerology, astronomy, mathematics, geometry, physics, alchemy and chemistry, to increase awareness in daily life. Tantra is a bridge between the soul and the universe. He believes in unity in the diversity and continuity of energy that goes through many transformations and always remains the same.

Tantra is therefore by its very nature non-dual, aimed at re-appropriation of the self, experimentation through the senses, celebration of life, a practical way and not of metaphysical abstractions, a way that does not impose renunciation or asceticism but which recognizes in desire the main force of manifestation of the divine in its human / incarnate dimension.

Tantra is the right system of knowledge, which when used properly, can provide tangible results and a high level of internal transformation. In the west is almost exclusively related to sexual relations. The communication media, which are attracted to the forbidden feeling in view of requests from the public, combine this practice of yoga with sex, and only as a series of techniques that increase pleasure.

Kamasutra also passed as an erotic / exotic text in the West, when in reality only a small part of this text - dating back to the 4th century BC. - is dedicated to sex positions: the treaty speaks above all of politics, economics, social norms and the sexual act is however considered as a divine union and an evolution of the human being. In tantric views, reality is perceived as a network in which the parts are united in all and where the whole is reflected in each part. Life itself is a tool for spiritual evolution, and therefore primary needs, including gender, are not only an important part of the effort to unite the mind, body and soul. Association which means awareness, love for oneself and authentic connection with oneself. Tantra is based on the principles of holy love.

Tantra in Sanskrit means "awareness-raising technique". Tantra is not a religion in the traditional sense, nor is it a philosophy or a mystical method based on a metaphysical concept, but an empirical instrument for those who are looking for something.

This is an experience-based technique in the real life field. Consciousness understood in this way covers all aspects of our lives, and in this field tantra is the only discipline where synthesis is made between seemingly opposite dimensions of pleasure and liberation.

The original tantra, also known as red or left hand, is associated with ancient matriarchal societies and has a female energy center. While tantra, called white or right hand and then created through Muslim infiltration, has its origins in Indian patriarchal societies such as the West today.

The difference between red tantra and white tantra is radical. The second tantra, white tantra, is based on static and lonely meditation, while red tantra is a practice where meditation is not just immobility and seriousness. In red tantra, meditation and holiness are experienced at every moment of their existence through listening deeply and paying attention to what is happening inside and outside us. Meditation occurs when dancing, running, hugging, eating, drinking, playing and talking.

There is a lot of confusion about what Tantra really is, and especially deliberate information due to the persecution that the original Tantra was targeted. Tantra carries with it the burden of false clichés, such as that of free sex. Unlike other disciplines that have been less polluted, Tantra is for many a kind of Yoga practice; for others an orgiastic practice and for still others a religion. In summary, the only true tantra is the one called Red. This does not mean that Tantric yoga, white and right-handed, cannot be useful tools; but if you practice them you should at least know that Tantra is not being done.

The origin

According to the almost unanimous opinion of scholars, the archaic nature of Red Tantra dates back to pre-Vedic cultures, to the very beginnings of Indian history, identifiable with the Harappan, Sindhu and other Dravidian populations who developed their civilization in the Indus valley. According to some in the third millennium BC these populations were widespread in a huge territory that went from Spain to the Ganges valley. Their precursors had settled in the Indus valley in Mehrgarh starting from 7000 BC. and their traces can be found up to 5500 BC.

Therefore, Dravidian populations, appeared there around 6000-5000 BC, had their apogee between 2300 and 1300 BC. and disappeared, rather quickly, in a 100-year period between 1900 and 1800 B.C. The reasons for the disappearance were attributed in the past to invasions of the Arii population from the north. Today there is a tendency to attribute it rather to a tectonic movement that caused the Aravali hills in northern Rajastan to rise, depriving river that supported the Dravidian civilization (the Ghaggar-Hakra) of most of its tributaries.

The Harappan population showed a marked interest in the arts and well-being. Their, was a matriarchal society, the most important central monument of their city, it was a large swimming pool; the element of water was fundamental in their society and there has already been a bathroom in every home. The woman is at the center of culture that focuses on the mother goddess. Female figures control the temple and worship with open arms and legs. The Harappans held a large bed in the center of the main hall of the house and practiced tantra. Their religion is closely related to the body, welfare, and sexuality.

In practice, white tantra is red tantra, but it is censored by all practices that moralists consider impossible to achieve. Today, white tantra, which is therefore a hoax from original tantra, is used commercially in the West. Almost all schools in Tantra practice White Tantra and therefore do not really teach Tantra.

True Tantra is the Way of reconnection with one's Self. It is the

Way; that of the discovery of our genotypic sexual energies that are manifested through the knowledge and practice of Origin Tantric.

How it came to the west

Regarding the sexual liberation of the 1960s and 1970s and the emancipation of women, some scientists and philosophers began to talk about tantra and tried to make it a practical approach also in the West, which made rituals more flexible and less obstructing.Currently emancipation allows women to get closer to the sexual world, although in western society it is still believed that sex is more masculine and feminine and cultural heritage and cultural heritage does not allow women to focus on that Tantra is a vehicle to reach well-being and a higher spirituality.

In the West today Tantra aims to draw two maps, one that indicates how to make the sexual experience spiritual and how to unite the earth with the sky, in a terrain where separation and judgment vanish and another map that brings you closer to the unknown sexual world (intended as unconditional love). So the Western world, where there are no schools and traditions because of Catholicism and the like and with which everything, must be thought out and tried. In the West, the sexual environment is a world that has been destroyed by taboo and religion for two millennia and is often only found in private clubs or on porn sites.

Tantra with all its erotic experiences is nothing more than a tool that opens up physical, emotional, and energetic space and awareness. Therefore, tantra is only red tantra. The way of liberation opens to the true expression of the self, which allows one to get out of the imagined and real dimensions of the matrix in which sexual energy is channeled mechanically for the wrong purpose. Sex and sexual energy are very different things.

The idea of sex is what in the imagination has settled during education, stories and commercial pornography; a program therefore, but so deeply rooted that individuals believe that it is precisely that pre-programmed way that sexual energy must be expressed. A program that is then gradually enhanced with the repetitive experiences that add up as memories.

Life energy, or commonly known as sexual energy, is the opposite of human essence in its origin; This is what we carry in our genes, but which is stated in fact in an unnatural way because of the formation contained in the matrix.

Over time, with the help of religious morality, the matrix selects sexual modalities that aim exclusively at reproduction ... because it is mechanically and aimed at penetration and orgasm to achieve goals; as if the whole miracle of contact between the body must be closed within minutes between two genital organs. Many people believe that they are sexually free because they do this much mechanical sex while in reality they are only slaves; Slaves became a trap in which true sexual energy was insulted and destroyed.

The real expression of sexual energy is flowers, sunsets or caresses every time we love something. And when this energy is released from the mechanism embedded in the mind, it becomes a ritual, a party, bodily connections, transcendence, healing energy, non-verbal communication, openness to trust between souls, breaking open mechanical schemes, projections into reality and into the world of imaginary love . Because love cannot be searched ... Love is the fruit of the tree of freedom.

It is therefore freedom to generate love and it is precisely by freeing oneself from the patterns that love is encountered.

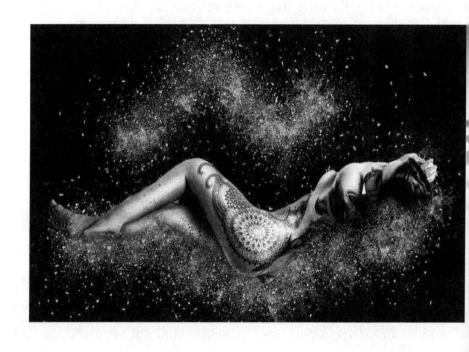

Chapter 2. Why everyone can benefit from Tantric sex

Tantric sex is a technique that allows you to reach a true state of ecstasy. A very pleasant orgasm that remains unforgettable. This experience allows you to experience intense emotions and feelings and to support your body and mind to free yourself from all boundaries. Let's find out what we know about tantric sex and why we should practice it.

- *Love*. For Tantra, love is very sacred. In fact, the woman will be a manifestation of the goddess Shakti, while the man will represent Lord Shiva on earth.

- *Sex*. For this reason, sex is a kind of sacred union of two gods: male and female energy merges into something beautiful and strong.

- *Body.* In tantric sex, it is important to be aware of your own body, to know your body and your partner's body. In particular, it is important to focus on points of contact with others without thinking about others.

- *Rhythm*. Tantra considers rhythm in sex to be very important. Partners must move in unison to release the energy in the pool level.

- **Breathing**. To stimulate excitement and pleasure, you must learn to breathe calmly. If breathing is difficult, the erogenous zone is not properly oxygenated and pleasure is not achieved.

- **Orgasm**. During tantric sex, pleasure must be maximized so that orgasm is delayed. In fact, the climax is not the final destination. It is important that the relationship lasts at least 35 minutes so that the pair's brain waves can be adjusted.

- **Traditional sex**. Tantra is different from traditional sex in many ways. First of all, this takes more time, also more orgasms and is far more diverse.

- **Couples.** Practicing tantric sex certainly has many benefits for couples. According to those who practice it, you can reach a good sentimental balance because it emphasizes the qualities and differences between men and women.

The Tantra Path consists of 3 steps:

1. Release your sexual energy - Not in the sense of unbridled sex, but in an affective sense: feeling at ease, reconnecting heart and sex, relaxing in the loving act and enjoying it to the fullest, distancing oneself from the many ideals that you have in your head (supermask, the always beautiful woman), cultivating an intimate communication with your partner, indulge in the most intimate sensations, share them in two and find pleasure in the temple of your body. If you see your inner monster on your face as soon as you reconnect with the raw energy of the first chakra, it is no longer a dream, it becomes very concrete: We begin to accept ourselves as we are, with fear, with Madness, feelings, desires, and deepest and deepest needs.

2. Increase pleasure - Many struggle with meditation, not because it comes from the East or because they are not disciplined enough, but because they cannot resist the joy that comes from it. We are all accustomed to certain limits of pleasure, and once we overcome them, we unwittingly implement strategies to reduce them again. For this reason, we cannot stand so open, loving, and vulnerable, even if the time of falling in love ends sooner or later. In tantra, on the other hand, we reconstruct the state in love, because it is the state that acts as a springboard to go into ecstasy, it is the key that more than any ascetic practice opens the door to the divine that everyone contains in himself. Let's look at sexuality from a new perspective: we can see that what we call "sex" is only 10% of what can be done with sex. We note that as self-taught (and all self-taught in terms of sex) we have a very limited view of pleasure.

Now we are ready to experience finer and finer aspects of sexuality, to experience it in a more peaceful and inner way, to try other forms of orgasm besides what we know to bring sexual energy (Kundalini) into the higher chakra to exchange energy between men and women that we don't even know about.

3. The next step of orgasm takes us to ecstasy - This is not about turning sex into "something purer or more spiritual" as the modern school of sexual oppression calls it in the new age, but about extending orgasm in the true meaning of the word. Ecstasy is nothing more than a bigger orgasm, an orgasm that fully rules us, which permeates the entire body, mind and body energy to bring us to our center, to emptiness, to full awareness, to extraordinary happiness.

When a man experiences a woman's part in himself and that woman is a man's part in himself, there may be what is called an inner marriage, which prepares us to get to know us and our partners without filters, without masks, without restrictions and in them the love of meditation spaces where a man and woman help each other to climb the chakra steps to join the sea of ecstatic orgasms and make love for hours ....

In tantra, sexuality is lived in a more internal way, sex, love and meditation are combined, the beacon of awareness is turned inwards and not outwards, one descends into the depth of one's soul, one travels in the territories of the psyche human, where the woman is usually more familiar. Therefore it is the woman who takes the lead in the tantric act: she guides times, rhythms, speed, pauses .....

The woman opens her body and the man penetrates her, the man opens his heart and the woman penetrates him with his love. Each one opens himself completely to the energy of the other and lets himself be impregnated until he is full, until he reaches the limits of his body-mind system and finds out what awaits him beyond ordinary consciousness.

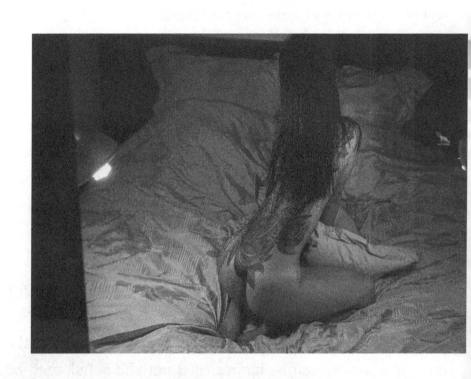

Chapter 3. The ancient secrets of Sexual energy

How do you determine your sexual energy? Can you define it? Can you recognize him? Can you see the strength and intensity? I am pretty sure that most people are a little shy and very modest in their sexual energy. This is a personal matter, and our world education teaches us to contain, isolate and limit only certain areas of sexual energy.

The result is that many people are inhibited and not only contain their sexual energy, but limit it, reduce it, turn it off. Through sanctions, not only related to sex. The ability to fully understand your own sexual energy is the ability to live alone, be in your own skin and body in the best possible way, to move in the world and to experience life with conscious acceptance for yourself and for yourself to live without any physical limitations and actions, limitation, or prejudice. This is a short way to be happy.

Have you ever thought about the power of sexual energy? On the other hand, it is thanks to him that our species lives and is able to reach it today. Very often, however, we cannot use sexual energy properly and much of it is lost.

Knowing how to use sexual energy in the right mood and how to channel it properly can also help to manage emotions and everyday life better. Sexual energy affects not only the many areas of partner relationships, intimate relationships and sexuality, but also our entire personality, all aspects of our lives. No one at school taught us the best way to regulate your sexuality. Blocked sexual energy is the main cause of sexuality that is not fulfilled.

Unfortunately, these energy blocks are consolidated in adulthood, and suppressed emotions make body strong and insensitive, inhibiting sexual energy and preventing a person from fully and satisfactorily undergoing his sexuality.

We live in a world where great emphasis is placed on sex, sexuality, presence and physical prowess. The fact is that all this happens from an almost exclusively "visual" point of view. They are the images that regulate our world and it is mainly through images that we manipulate our minds. The winner is the product, the politician or character who, when described or described - even if only in words - is defined through images. "Imaginative" words are said, which recreate images in our mind. Sensuality also passes through images and is maintained in the image only.

The male and lady sexual energy

As a primary detail it would be essential to underline how often a big part of our sexual electricity is wasted. In guys this takes place by using ejaculation, in ladies at the side of menstruation. for this it'd be necessary to understand the way to stability what is loss of sexual strength, earlier than additionally being capable of control it within the proper manner.

There are unique strategies that allow not handiest to reduce the fatigue that can result from having "wasted" sexual energy, but additionally to use it properly. Por instance, guys can discover ways to control ejaculation while not having to surrender orgasm, accordingly having access to pride while not having to lose the saved electricity.

Inside the same way, ladies lose plenty of strength whilst the cycle arrives. They may be also located mentally exhausted, and this is a demonstration of lack of sexual energy. Unluckily in lots of instances women discover their femininity with menstruation, no longer understanding that it must be unbiased of the menstrual cycle, which is often best a supply of discomfort and ache for many ladies.

Having available again that sexual energy that would otherwise be lost in these situations will allow you to have more resources to be able to direct towards your creativity and to areas of your life that could significantly benefit from it. This is the passion capability, magnetism, power, sexuality, creativity expressiveness, that this person has innately in his nature as a human being. This applies to both adults and kids.

Sexual strength has been part of us because our introduction / thought, and it acts in us from the intrauterine ranges at some point of pregnancy. The balance of internal and outside float of this strength, regardless from the individual's age, from his faith or from his way of life, it is of essential significance for his popular health, and specially for physical health. Living a harmonious and balanced inner relationship, free and loving with the one's sexual energy means being free from mental forms of judgment, guilt, repression, and negative emotions such as, for example, insecurity, fear, non-acceptance, a sense of inferiority, shame, the need to demonstrate and give to get something in return, devaluation of your body.

Yogic know-how suggests that this electricity is liable for the formation of the child within the womb, and after start it stays rolled up at the bottom of the backbone for you to preserve the strength intact in stasis till death, whilst it unwinds and returns to its supply.

However, Kundalini can also deviate or unwind from the base of the spine as a result of certain spiritual practices, or in response to life events. When this takes place, it can be moved little by little, unrolling like a snake, or quickly and explosively, related to the intestine, coronary heart or head. This occasion can be unexpected and chaotic, frightening or comfortable, and generally triggers months and years of recent sensations and changes in the person that awakens this electricity.

You can clearly perceive the balance of the body moving and failing, and it takes time to adapt. Awakening Kundalini is a practice considered in the East very significant for the spiritual realization of each individual, but it is rarely recognized as such in Western traditions, and perhaps for this reason Western peoples are more easily affected by energy or physical problems related to the malfunction of this energy.

References to Kundalini are found in lots of yogic and tantric traditions, in buddhism, taoism, the magical gnostic culture and a few native american teachings, as well as indigenous societies.

The photograph of a snake that crosses the complete frame i recalled in the esoteric art of many cultures, as well as the capability to intensify and increase the body's strength, which has been explored for hundreds of years.

The liberty to live your sexual electricity has nothing to do with the free sex meant as with out policies or performed with all o us, without standards choice, as it is not just about the liberty o body expression of sexuality. Our sexual energy is our recharge of life par excellence, and there we are many misunderstandings about its correct use and its real nature, created both from religious and social culture in the various historical periods, up to ours days.

True sexual freedom allows you to fully enjoy the pleasure in al areas of life, allows us to express the true nature of ourselves exactly as we are, it allows the liberation of our creativity and its manifestation in all its forms, which are not closely related to artistic forms.

In truth, we imply a each day creativity, which begins from small things, by way of get to the pinnacle ... A creativity that allows you to create each day
constantly what makes you feel full, satisfied, mild, completely

satisfied, thankful for lifestyles and for the whole thing it is able to provide, in keeping with your desires.

How to start forfeiting sexual energy

Given these assumptions, one might think that to accumulate sexual energy at best, it is sufficient for men to have a vasectomy and for women to take a birth control pill. This type of reasoning, in reality, is completely incorrect, as these remedies negatively affect the body, its rhythms and also its naturalness. Otherwise, however, one should try to acquire awareness of one's sexual energy and learn first to know it and then not to waste it, without external interventions. In this regard, there are exercises and techniques that can be used.

Techniques for controlling sexual energy

Depending on the cultures and religions present in the various countries of the world, the idea of sexual energy changes, and also what the approaches to its correct management can vary. In particular, for the Chinese, the use of sexual energy should take place precisely to increase that of the body, to positively influence creativity and to help in everyday life. At the same time, the correct management of this energy will help, always for the techniques used since ancient times in China, also to enjoy the best of one's sexuality, which will no longer be animalistic and uncontrolled, but will be a moment of full expression for the human being.

Examples of techniques used in China for the control and use of sexual energy are tantric applications. These are often revealed only by the teacher to his students, and can be applied within groups that follow a certain philosophy of life. Even Indian philosophies often deal with talking about sexuality, and in particular its sacred character. For Indians, in fact, sex was never a particular taboo, but they immediately understood the importance of the correct use of sexual energy, so as not to waste that present in the body.

Sexual energy, in Hinduism, often has two "colors", male and female, also represented by the same deities that are present in their pantheon. The union of these two energies determines perfection, but it must always be carried out with a certain awareness. Concept of Kundalini as sexual energy belongs to Hinduism, and now to Indian culture in general.

It can be understood as a life force, which remains dormant in many human beings, to awaken when the conditions are favorable, or when efforts are made to perform precise techniques. The Kundalini can, if released, begin to flow from the base of the back to the head along what is an energy channel which corresponds to the spine and which is called Sushumna Nadi. To have the ability, but, to manipulate this sort of electricity it will be important no longer handiest to recognise the way to awaken it, however additionally a way to channel it and the way to control it better.

Consequently, there are sporting activities that will let you intervene at the blocks related to sexual electricity, or on its waste, and on the management of these two components. The sporting activities, which belong each to the style of Kundalini yoga, and to other strategies constantly coming from the indian heritage, act on the first chakra, that of the basis, as a way to intervene on what can be the limits that do not allow you to freely express one's sexual energy, now not handiest in the real dating, however additionally as creative strength.

Physical exercises for sexual strength
To discover ways to manage sexual electricity it will likely be important, first of all, to collect a whole awareness of it. For this, exceptional types of body notion sports could be accomplished. simply in Yoga, it will likely be possible to start through paying attention to your very own respiration and to what are the sensations that derive from a deep and managed respiratory.

Sports will then be done in order to involve chakras, power centers of frame, and in an effort to permit, already on a physical degree, to understand the electricity found in these electricity facilities and alongside the channels that join them. At a meditative level, it'll then be viable to first visualize the energy and manage it, then, consciously, directing it, keeping it or the use of it.

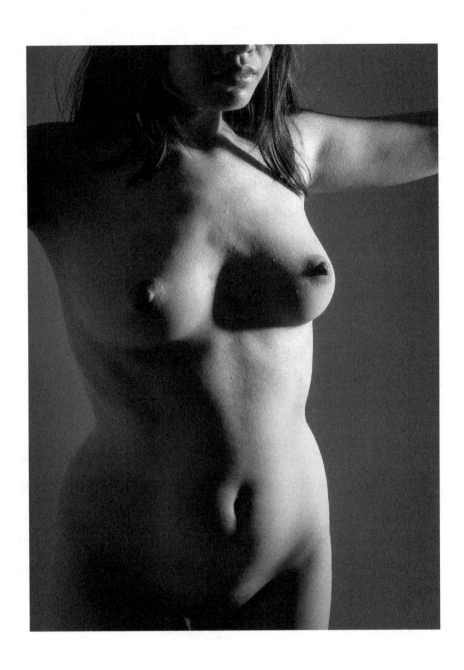

Chapter 4. The 7 Chakras of vitality and life balance

You've got probably heard of chakras as a minimum once in your existence. The 7 chakras are in fact key factors inside the philosophy of yoga on the grounds that they're very crucial electricity centers found in our frame. In this chapter we are able to see in element what chakras are, how they work and a way to awaken them with the exercise of yoga and meditation, which will gain severa psychophysical blessings. Chakra is a sanskrit word which means wheel, disk or circle. Chakras are our essential factors and represent the electricity centers of our frame that have the task of absorbing our crucial strength (prana) and distributing it externally.

In our frame 74 chakras are counted however of those best 7 are the fundamental or principal chakras. Every of these 7 chakras is positioned at a selected factor in our frame and they may be distributed among the head and the bottom of the spine Although we've got given them a spatial area, the chakras are not part of our physical frame however of our subtle frame, that is our emotional part.

The energy chakras, also are represented with lotus vegetation seen from above. Exactly for that reason they also can take the name of padma, because of this "lotus". Every lotus representing a chakra additionally has a different wide variety of petals and a unique coloration and incorporates different elements, together with a mantra, a letter of the sanskrit alphabet at the petals or a symbol with a specific meaning.

Each chakra is also related to particular factors, which include colorings, sounds, stones and so forth. After this premise, you're possibly questioning, "why are chakras so critical to us?" It is quite simple.

The chakras are essential factors in our body because they're robust lively facilities that join the body and the psyche together. Whilst the chakras are open, strength can drift freely, with tremendous results for both the mind and the body. However while the chakras are closed, the energy can not float, forming a blockage that causes terrible repercussions each bodily and emotionally. Because of this, it's far very important that chakras constantly stay open and i can give an explanation for to you shortly a way to do that.

The origins of the 7 chakras
Inside the history of yoga, the oldest text in which we speak of the 7 chakras that we realize nowadays is the kubjikāmata

tantra, an critical file of hindu culture. But, there are nonetheless more ancient texts wherein reference is made to the chakras, this is the vedas, sacred texts of the indian scriptures Already on the time it became understood that in the body there are strength points that would be opened and advanced via the exercise of yoga and meditation.

The culture of the chakras has therefore been passed down from era to generation, via the written texts and the teachings of the masters to their disciples, until they have got become so fundamental inside the philosophy of yoga to attain us.

How the 7 chakras work

The chakras are 7 power centers located in our body located among the top and the decrease part of the spine and are:

Muladhara - Earth or root chakra

Svadhisthana - Water or sacral chakra

Manipura - Fire or solar plexus chakra

Anahata - Heart chakra

Visuddha - Purifying or throat chakra

Ajna - Chakra of light or third eye

Sahasrara - Crown chakra

These energy centers have the task of receiving energy and redistributing it through the nadis, of the fate of channels connected to the backbone which have the task of transporting energy to the rest of the body. Our goal will therefore always be to maintain the right opening of our chakras, in a balanced way, so that energy can flow smoothly without having energy blocks (closed chakras) or an energy overload (chakras too open). Both of these situations can in fact lead to both mental and physical malaise.

Since the chakras are connected to the nerve ganglia and endocrine glands, the closure of the chakras and the consequent energy block that derives from them can cause a state of internal crisis and mental and physical discomfort as well as the onset of pathologies to the organs connected to those glands. When a chakra is awakened and then opened, we become more aware of ourselves and develop specific psychophysical benefits.

The chakras are also not disconnected from each other, but have a strong influence on each other, especially as regards chakras close to each other. This means that opening or closing a chakra can positively or negatively affect adjacent chakras.

So, every chakra has a precise color and a representing stone.

Stones and crystals have beneficial influences and used in combination with the chakras they also increase their effect. I you are looking for a set of chakra stones to use during your meditation, you can find it here. Now that we apprehend what chakras are and the way they work and after staring at how crucial their stability is, we come to a vital question:

"How to discover if chakras are blocked? And the way do you open them?"

Later, when I describe the character chakras separately, i will also give you examples to apprehend if one or extra of your chakras are unbalanced. When a chakra is simply too closed or too open, in fact, there are some bodily, emotional and intellectual imbalances that exercise or meditation will help you resolve. By way of aligning the chakras, a balance can also be received to your frame, in order that the thoughts and body can stay in unison, with all the blessings and high-quality consequences that derive from it.

The 7 chakras
Now that we realize what chakras are and how they work, let's take a better observe every man or woman chakra!

1 - *Muladhara: the root chakra*

First Chakra - Muladhara. The word Muladhara comes from Sanskrit and literally means "support of the base". This chakra is placed at the bottom of the backbone, inside the perineum. It's far the chakra this is connected to the legs and is consequently a image of the earth and all this is stable and solid. Because of this it is also the chakra of all the toughest elements of the body, consisting of the nails, bones and tooth.

The basis chakra or first chakra symbolizes balance, self-self assurance and protection and is connected to our survival. When it's balanced we sense confident, quite, happy and capable of stay the existing second, complete of enthusiasm and geared up to plot our future. It's far in truth crucial to have strong roots on which to relaxation our whole lifestyles, just as the roots for the survival of a tree or the foundations for constructing a strong house are essential.

While the primary chakra is blocked, we will sense misplaced, apathetic, disheartened and unsafe in ourselves. we can by no means feel happy in area and could have a tendency to change homes or fatherland often. Even our body is stricken by the blockage of this chakra: we are able to feel tired and exhausted, we are able to have issues with our enamel, kidneys and our joints.

When, on the other hand, it is too open, opposite feelings are triggered, such as a strong attachment to material goods and the past, without being able to live in the present moment. W oppose change and develop a total lack of fear or excessive fear which can lead us to get into very risky situations or the inability to enjoy the beauty of life.

The way to stability the first chakra

To stability the chakras you ought to by no means pretend to be what you are not. For instance, you don't need to pretend to be satisfied on the way to align it, but on the contrary, if you contro to rebalance it, you may start to experience happy.

There are numerous physical activities, positions and visualizations that you can do to release the primary chakra. The primary component i propose you to do is to discover a quiet region where you could be immediately in touch with the earth like a grove or a garden. Even the house garden is quality Practice positions that inspire your contact with the earth inclusive of vrksasana, the placement of the tree, or tadasana the placement of the mountain.

Additionally do visualization activities. Take a seat at the ground with your legs crossed and your again straight. Now visualize the roots that start out of your body to go deep into the ground. As the roots sink, they will bring all the terrible energies you have got accumulated. While you sense geared up, call the roots in the direction of you, that allows you to go back collectively with the tremendous electricity of the earth.

2 - Svadhisthana: the splenic chakra

Second Chakra - The Svadhisthana. Continuing the journey of ascent of the kundalini, the second chakra we find is the splenic chakra or water chakra. Unlike the first, which indicates stability, this chakra is associated with liquids, therefore with letting it flow, with flowing, with the ability to change.

The second chakra is the fulcrum between body and soul. It's miles placed inside the lower stomach, simply below the navel, and is the chakra of emotions, spontaneity, creativity, pleasure and sexuality. While the water chakra is blocked, feelings are maximum affected. In truth, we've sturdy temper swings, we're full of anger, guilt and shame and we're problem to panic attacks. The look for intercourse turns into a mere bodily stimulus however without related to emotions.

This inevitably results in unsatisfactory tales with you companions. Physically, issues and pathologies can occur in the lower stomach region, along with kidney stones and dysfunctions of the reproductive machine and menstrual cycle in addition to what concerns the go with the flow of fluids consisting of the circulatory system or the bladder. If second one chakra is too open, a search for immediate however ephemera delight and fulfillment occurs, growing emotional or food alcohol, drug or intercourse addictions.

How to rebalance the second chakra

To rebalance the second one chakra you'll need to work in you feelings and creativity. All-spherical yoga practice will help you examine and control your feelings. Respiration is also very vita to rebalance the splenic chakra. Just like a fluid, in reality, you'll have with a view to permit the air you breathe for the duration of your body glide.

 # 3 - Manipura: the solar chakra

Third Chakra. The third chakra, i.e. the solar chakra or fire chakra, is located in the solar plexus, the part of the abdomen that is located between the diaphragm and the navel. If the primary chakra is attached to balance and the second to flowing, the third chakra is the union of these two elements, this is mild, energy, warmth and while it's nicely balanced we feel active, certain of ourselves , sturdy and masters of ourselves.

We are not fearful of others' judgments and we continually know a way to address the scenario and we don't have any problem in coping with ourselves and our feelings. It's far related to digestive system and digestion, which "devours" food just as a fire devour what it reveals in its direction.

When the third chakra is unbalanced we can be aware many terrible signs and symptoms, each bodily and mentally, in particular associated with our safety and our digestive system. When it's far too closed, in reality, we word the onset of lack of confidence, low vanity, introversion and a strong experience of inadequacy in all conditions. At the bodily level, however, troubles which includes liver issues, nausea, ulcer, gastritis, difficulty in digestion and celiac disorder get up.

Troubles also can appear whilst this chakra is just too open, making someone appear very boastful, competitive, all too self-confident, in regular search for strength and who usually feels the want to self-celebrate to hide their defeats and their own. insecurities.

A way to rebalance this chakra

To rebalance the Manipura chakra you may exercise all the positions related to the stomach, inclusive of the navasana, the placement of the boat, or the parivrtta trikonasana, the location of the circled triangle.

4 - Anahata: the heart chakra

Fourth Chakra. The Anahata heart chakra is the most central one. It unites the higher chakras, more spiritual and representing elements that are on the ground, with the lower ones, more material and golden.

The Anahata also represents the air, which unites the earth with the sky. the fourth chakra is therefore a real hyperlink among the above and below, between the ground and the non secular, and this is additionally proven by using the two triangles inner, one with the end pointing upwards, indicating the sky, and one with the end down, to suggest the earth. The fourth chakra is intently related to the lungs and respiration.

Whilst it's open we are capable of love unconditionally, showing ourselves beneficent with others, being concerned and heartfelt.

However we are not completely dependent on others and we can also love ourselves and our life.

Physically, the air manages to go into fluidly into our lungs, loaded with oxygen, that's transported to the relaxation of body by using a functional circulatory system. If the fourth chakra closes, the resulting problems are associated with the affective sphere. We are incapable of loving ourselves to start with and consequently also the ones around us. We come to be cold and apathetic, always wary and circumspect because we generally tend no longer to accept as true with anybody.

If it opens an excessive amount of, but, our interest will cognizance exclusively on others to divert interest from ourselves. However it will no longer be a selfless love: we can try to derive the greatest quantity of benefits from a relationship, without the goal of giving something in go back.

How to rebalance the fourth chakra

The Asanas that assist reopen the fourth chakra are all those wherein the chest is the protagonist, inclusive of anahatasana or dhanurasana, and all breathing techniques, such as pranayama.

5 - *Vishuddha: the throat chakra*

Fifth Chakra. As the name indicates, the Vishuddha chakra i located right at the base of the throat and is connected t communication, both with others and with ourselves, and th emotions that derive from it.

The color of this chakra is blue and symbolizes transparency When this chakra is open, in fact, you can express yoursel clearly and limpidly, with tact, without offending. Your voice i calm and relaxed, you can listen to others and you can alway express what you think and let yourself go.

The opening of the fifth chakra also brings great creativity which is a very powerful means of expressing yourself. Ou social relationships are pleasant and relaxed, we are intensel interested in others with understanding and without judging.

Our concentration is likewise very high. For the reason tha we're very predisposed to listening, learning additionally wil become speedy and powerful. At the opposite, the closure of thi chakra ends in failure to specific oneself nicely or to pa attention to others. We are unable to say no, we feel extremel shy and clumsy and we are no longer able to express ou creativity, either through words or through artistic disciplines.

All this results in a situation of profound discomfort that in the end will make us near so much in ourselves that we do no longer want or even be afraid of being with other human beings. Pointless to mention, our social relationships will inevitably collapse.

Even on a bodily level we are able to run into troubles, initially to the thyroid, but also to respiratory and related organs. Malaise which includes asthma, bronchitis, mouth sores, speech problems however additionally ear infections and ear pains will seem.

While the chakra is just too open and works an excessive amount of, we turn out to be talkative, without ever being attentive to what others are telling us. But, what we are saying is not what we virtually suppose however our conversations can be primarily based on lies and manipulations. We also experience overconfident and don't accept grievance, even when it comes from the people we love.

The way to rebalance the fifth chakra
When it is unbalanced, what we want to do is carry out our

creativity and discover ways to admire silence and listening.

It does not count number when you have a creative block. Try to combat it through portray, writing, dancing or singing, even supposing the result will no longer be the fine! the crucial aspect is so one can allow move of your feelings.

You could additionally exercise asanas that affect the neck and shoulders, inclusive of matsyasana, also known as the placement of the fish. I additionally suggest you to do meditation, concentrating deeply for your breathing.

6 - Ajna: the third eye chakra
Sixth Chakra. In the 6th chakra we keep upwards within the direction of the kundalini, as much as the penultimate chakra: the third eye chakra.

The third eye chakra is placed within the head, among the eyebrows, and is the image of instinct and imaginative and prescient past appearances and past even truth itself.

It's far unavoidably linked to the eyes but additionally to the brow, temples, brain and spinal cord. On this chakra are related all opposites and all dualities, including male and lady, purpose and instinct, shape and substance, body and mind, precise and awful. A the third eye sees what exists besides those concepts, dissolving the dualities to get to peer the actual reality.

If the waft of electricity that passes thru this 5th chakra is not blocked, we song into our higher self. We become intuitive, aware, focused and distinctly perceptive. we're able to visualize mind and snap shots, empathy is amplified and we will control to understand what different people think.

We see the world for what it is, in its power and in its spirituality, with expertise and without prejudice. We can understand the essence of what surrounds us, seeing past what we bodily appearance with our eyes. While ajna is blocked, we end up egocentric, cynical, materialistic, bloodless and calculating. We most effective agree with what we see with our eyes and we can not understand what exists past. We can no longer dream or plan our future, we become insensitive and detached, without the ability to stay focused for long on something.

On a physical level, the head will be affected: headache, migraine, tiredness, insomnia, neurosis, pain in the eyes and even blindness. But the sixth chakra can also be too open and in this case in addition to physical pain we become manic, self-celebrating and we tend to blame others for our faults too. It is therefore important that the sixth chakra is always balanced to maintain inner serenity and a stable relationship with others.

How to rebalance the sixth chakra

Want to rebalance the third eye chakra? The meditation is crucial. In fact, through meditation we can put ourselves in communication with ourselves and with the energy that is around us. Even the practice of yoga undoubtedly brings you closer to this goal.

It is also important to practice pranayama to learn how to benefit from our breathing. In addition to yoga and meditation, to rebalance the sixth chakra you can carry out activities that stimulate creativity or immerse yourself in nature, paying attention to the small details of life and contemplating the beauties that are around us every day, such as a sunset or a starry sky.

7 - *Sahasrara: the crown chakra*

Seventh Chakra. Eventually we arrive at 7th chakra, the best, the ultimate one that reaches the kundalini on this ascent: the crown chakra. About this chakra, Osho Rajneesh stated:

The moment your energy is released from the sahasrara [...] you are no longer a man. At that point you don't belong to this Earth; you have become divine. Sahasrara is the special chakra of liberation and knowledge. It is not located inside the physical body, but above, above the pinnacle. It is connected to the strength of the universe, to the connection with the divine, to enlightenment. Folks who reach this degree could have understood the mysteries of existence, which include birth and death.

This chakra is represented through a lotus with one thousand petals, a symbolic range that indicates infinity. Its power will dissolve your ego into the entire and flip us into idea. The outlet of the 7th chakra will come up with know-how, properly-being, tranquility and happiness. You will be affected person, know-how and compassionate. But what happens if the strength glide of the 7th chakra is blocked? When it is blocked, we will now not be capable of cultivate our spirituality. We will consequently feel apathetic, discouraged, unwilling to live, depressed.

If, however, it is too open, we are able to then be attached to unimportant matters, fabric goods and electricity, overwhelmed by means of lack of knowledge and dissatisfaction and we will

continually experience aggravating, arrogant, impatient
Additionally at the physical aircraft we will suffer and accuse
exhaustion, intellectual confusion, depression, apathy till i
outcomes in psychosis and schizophrenia.

How to rebalance the 7th chakra

The positions that help us rebalance the seventh chakra are
people who stimulate the top of the pinnacle, together with
sirsasana or sasangasana, however also padmasana, additionally
known as lotus function, a good way to assist you find awareness
for meditation.

We've got come to the give up of this lengthy and charming
adventure to find out the 7 chakras.
Collectively we noticed what chakras are, how they work and
why it's so critical that they're constantly open and aligned.
Retaining the stability of the 7 chakras will help you live a
complete and peaceful existence, acquiring an ideal courting
both with yourself and with the human beings round you,
growing know-how, beauty and serenity, until you attain a deep
peace and harmony with the electricity of the universe.

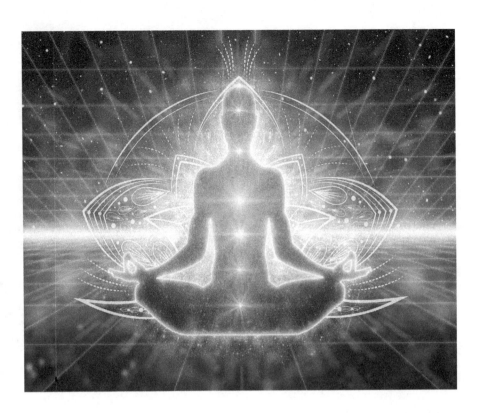

Chapter 5. Understanding sexual needs of your partner

Intercourse starts with interest to the partner: Recognition of the other's needs through emotional validation, listening and affection would increase sexual desire in long-lasting couples.

All the experts agree in confirming that sexual harmony is very important for maintaining a happy, peaceful and lasting relationship. Maintaining harmony and sexual desire is, on the other hand, the more difficult the more stable the relationship tends to become. The popular saying of marriage "tomb of love" is proof of this according to the "vox populi vox dei" principle.

The daily routine, job and, above all, the arrival of children who demand interest and are placed first within the care and attention, cause relegating intercourse rather low on the size of priorities. Inevitably, life in commonplace suffers and ends up turning into monotonous if not unacceptable. As many surveys show, a number of which conducted with first rate care and reliability, maximum married couples file have sex-related troubles.

In the first place two causes closely related to each other: intercourse practiced automatically, which considerably reduces delight and which necessarily ends in a lower inside the frequency of intercourse which is the second problem indicated in the survey. Yet it need to be remembered that regardless of every day issues, nothing can replace intercourse, the dearth of which, both in phrases of frequency and libido, remains the primary motive for the failures.

Consistent with an american studies conducted among stable couples between the ages of nineteen and forty nine, as a minimum eighty% of guys say that intercourse is the most critical element of marriage and that they would love their wives to be greater interested and more informal in have sex.

Amongst girls, on the other hand, handiest 12% of respondents stated they felt satisfied after having sexual intercourse with their spouse or associate. As for the frequency of intercourse, less than 50% of solid couples stated that they had at least one intercourse consistent with week. The most negative data relates to the fantasy item. For 80% of ladies, the relationship is predictable and unimaginative.

Intercourse in a pair relationship is one of the fundamental elements because it acts as a glue to hold the 2 halves together. It consequently represents a kind of thermometer to assess the diploma of intensity and closeness between two partners. The presence of intercourse regardless of the disagreements is a sign of a few shape of complicity which could make a dating preserve up despite the fact that there are evident difficulties; at the opposite, the total absence shows that the two people are shifting away and also disengaging in other areas (talk, sharing of interests, mutual support ...).

In order for the sex to be completely excellent for both members of the couple, every have to chance establishing up totally to the partner, making himself prone, sharing instead profound and strictly personal fantasies and desires. This openness is found out simplest if inside the dating all of us feels valued, favored, vital, loved, established and revered unconditionally.

However, the way ladies and men conceive intercourse is distinctive. the expectations concerning the accomplice in phrases of intercourse trade in keeping with the type of belonging. whilst the expectations of one or both partners are unnoticed, the relationship starts to be lived with dissatisfaction, unhappiness and frequent misunderstandings.

What are the expectancies that males and females usually have with appreciate to couple intimacy? They're exactly one of a kind from 5 parameters:

1. *Attentional focus:* most men tend to give importance to physical contact and visual stimuli (looking or imagining the partner). The response time to the erotic stimulus is short, within a few minutes. Once the sexual stimulus has produced excitement, the man is ready to have sexual intercourse. The importance that men attach to sex is greater than women; it's a priority. The woman approaches sex differently. It essentially seeks relationship and emotional involvement rather than physical and sexual contact in itself.

2. *Erotic stimuli:* excitement, preceded by external or internal stimulation, leads the man to an erection and the woman to vaginal lubrication. While the man is stimulated by specific aspects of his partner and therefore eroticizes through sight, (real or imaginary or fantasy stimulus), touch, the sense of smell the woman is instead stimulated by overall aspects such as attitudes, the actions and way of speaking of your partner. The woman does not just give relevance to the physical act but looks at the person as a whole to feel attracted.

3. *Needs:* the man feels the need to be respected, to enjoy the

admiration of his woman, to feel that it is necessary while th woman is looking for a partner who shows her understanding love and dedicates time even during foreplay. The former need a self-reported need to feel confirmed in his ego, the latter need emotional support and protection.

4. *Sexual response:* in man, it is acyclic, which means that h can get excited and have an intimate relationship at any tim and anywhere. Conversely, the woman's response is cyclical; sh goes through moments when she is more interested in sex and others when she can do without it. A man quickly gets a erection while the woman is much slower in reaching the plateau or the stage that precedes orgasm and where the level o excitement reaches its climax. Another difference lies in the fac that while the man during sex manages to focus only or performance, the woman is more easily distracted by externa stimuli (what happens around, from children, from noises).

5. *Orgasm:* it is the phase in which pleasure reaches its peak and there is a temporary loss of contact with external reality Here are the most significant differences between men and women. The former has a sexual release or orgasm in relatively short times and is physically observable while the female one is not obvious and can therefore be simulated.

The first, most vital step to stimulating sexual preference is communication.

Communicating does no longer mean clearly "speakme" and should no longer be limited handiest to the request for sex. We additionally communicate, every now and then in particular, via our personal behavior, gestures and attentions. Wives in dressing robes and curlers and husbands in vests and knickers, as a great deal as joke stereotypes, are the maximum common example of bad communication that not handiest does no longer produce sexual stimuli, but indicates an apparent disinterest in one's partner.

It's vital to stimulate and preserve the hobby alive with non-stop attention in the direction of the companion, as an example, in no way letting compliments, caresses and diverse seductions be lacking. Chiefly, one should not be ashamed or scared of making one's sexual dreams and fantasies explicit. Understand that all of us have it and communicate about it delicately but without conditioning, without worry of transgressing, being judged or being conditioned with the aid of ethical or instructional taboos.

One of the stumbling blocks on which the sexual desires of couples break is precisely due to the inability to talk about their sexual needs and fantasies. Confessing one's thoughts makes it easier. Feel free to make clear what you don't prefer. An attitude, a position, a movement, the important thing is to say it.

There may be no want to be ashamed of sexual goals and wishes, because there may be simply nothing to be ashamed of.

Sex is lovely and special due to the fact it's miles one of the moments of best freedom for both sexes. There aren't any rules, there aren't any limits, there may be no fear. the main rule is to allow pass and deliver unfastened rein to each fantasy and test. Absolutely everyone has something to learn and new pleasures to attempt, irrespective of their bedroom revel in.

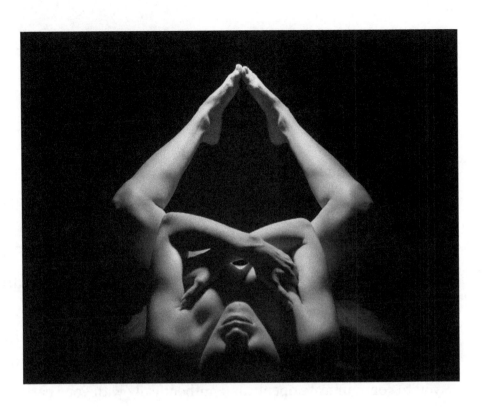

Chapter 6. How to prepare an unforgettable bedroom erotic experience

Tantric intercourse is a unique enjoy, a philosophy of life, a doctrine that has little to do with the sexual positions of the kamasutra. It permits the body and mind to lose themselves and to experience extreme, deep sensations of real bliss.

In ultra-modern society, where sexuality is experienced extra with the head than with the body, tantric intercourse teaches the importance of slowness, attention, naturalness and complicity, all traits that deepen intimacy and growth passion , permitting you to communicate openly and authentically with your partner. Not like conventional intercourse, in tantric sex it's miles important to pass over the anxiety of orgasm, overall performance, result and instead you need to learn how to revel in eroticism in its entirety, from sounds to breaths, up to movements.

Tantric sex is suggested only for people who are especially near due to the fact it is a more mental than physical exercise that brings out all the mental problems and motivations that underlie a dating. At the identical time, it's a exercise that fights routine and allows you to create a deep, passionate connection, a actual spiritual illumination. To stand it inside the fine way, to begin with you must not be afraid to attempt something new. handiest with the mind and with the open coronary heart will it's feasible to reach general leisure. Finally, you should determine to commit as a minimum one hour a week to your sexuality, even while you are tired or careworn. Tantric sex is in truth able to invigorating the frame and making it more potent and extra lively. Further, the atmosphere could be very essential to attain the climax of pride: the bedroom have to be a magical area, a temple of affection, a actual feast of the senses. It's far therefore top to beautify the mattress with pillows, blankets, plants, incense and even some fruit and beverages. at this point, you can loosen up, doing away with any blockage or tension that stops the frame from experiencing deep and excessive pride.

In tantric sex, it's far essential to take a seat in the front of the associate and meditate with him, connecting one's breath and coronary heart with that of the alternative. Although it is able to appear a ordinary practice, once you attempt tantra positions, the delight will develop into a real bliss. Tantric sex is a field additionally open to homosexuals, who can exercise a sensual erotic massage for his or her partner. Such an intimate second manages to rediscover your frame and gain excessive pride.

Homosexuality within the east has in no way been considered taboo and it's far precisely for this reason that the sort o passionate and excessive sexual practice is open to all sorts o gender.

Whether you are romantic or extraordinarily passionate, there i no place more intimate than the bedroom for the perfect evenin; for 2 having tantric sex. And in case you are thinking of ar alternative appointment or a spicy after dinner, better prepar the space in the best way, making it welcoming and inviting.

Because it's all about creating the proper ecosystem: the histor; music, the proper soft lighting fixtures and in the middle he, th mattress, absolutely the protagonist, protected with fashion anc a touch of sensuality, without forgetting the good flavor.

Ready to add a few pepper for your bedroom? check m suggestions now to find out how to show it into the best lov nest!

Do not disturb
The idea is to create an intimate and reserved space inside th room that most of all is intended for privacy and relaxation. Fo a really comfortable and cozy atmosphere, the four-poster bed i

the perfect choice. Alternatively, you could always play with fabrics that come down from the ceiling, creating a soft and sensual play of light.

Yes to order, no to technology

Nothing is greater sexy and inviting than a clean and tidy room. Eliminate any useless odds and ends, placed garments in their vicinity as well as books and numerous items: even the eye (and the nose) need its component and a room with light tones, free of needless furniture and sparkling air safe intimacy and luxury helping to "let move". Identical is going with tech devices: tvs, computers and electronic devices have to be left out of the bed room to concentrate all of the energies on the couple warding off distractions.

Opposite to popular notion, a chaotic erotic chamber filled with rose petals can inhibit the companion, inflicting him to shut in on himself and also cause him overall performance tension. For this reason, it's far better to choose a sober and orderly look, which shall we the entirety "come by itself" without any constraints in any respect. White sheets and blankets with darkish or red decorations, or pastel shades, are best for making the bed seem smooth, white however nevertheless appetizing. Avoid overly colored covers and complete of decorations. Blankets and duvets are available at a fee among 10 euros and

90 euros.

Gifts

A very original idea is to make your boyfriend find a gift at the foot of the bed, to be discarded together perhaps with some background of jazz music. Among the gifts to be made, sex toys are very popular, small objects to be used together to make the night together even more hot and fiery. Before making such a gift, however, one must have a lot of intimacy with one's partner, to avoid being disappointed. If, knowing the partner, he will not appreciate, you can choose to buy a gift he has long wanted: a smartwatch (starting from 17 euros), a pair of shoes (starting from 30 euros), a book (starting from 5 euros), etc; taking the opportunity of Valentine's Day to give him an object he needed.

Read protagonist

Imposing, tall, soft and comfortable: the bed is certainly the protagonist of your room and deserves a central position of all respect, so as to attract attention becoming completely irresistible. His choice depends on your style, but in general, prefer it quite comfortable, wide and inviting.

The perfect linen

Sheets, rugs and curtains speak volumes about your person and bed linen, too, will have to make a difference. You prefer quality fabrics, soft and pleasant in contact with the skin, the choice of shades is yours, as long as they are perfectly in tune with each other and not too eccentric and particular to distract attention to the most beautiful. Don't forget plenty of blankets and pillows to create pleasant layers of comfort and intimacy.

Pre-evening romantic
The bed is not the only romantic corner of the room and if you are thinking of an unforgettable moment at home, you just need to belong to the foot of the bed by decorating the space around you with flowers and candles. Whether it's enjoying an alternative dinner, giving good news or warming the atmosphere, passion will skyrocket.

Candlelight
Usually lights inside the room to create the best atmosphere for your evenings as a pair. And when you have a crackling fire to cheer you up on less warm nights, you will have accomplished perfection. As an alternative to candles, you could constantly create the right environment with small lights to be placed around the bed: they make the room greater intimate and sensual and are decidedly romantic. Candles are absolutely inevitable inside the design of the erotic bedroom. The lighting

fixtures in question, in truth, control to create an ideal suffused surroundings to whet any kind of fable. Anyways, in case you are organizing a night meeting, it's far better that you avoid lighting fixtures the room handiest with candles, so as not to hazard developing a macabre surroundings. it is right, consequently, which you additionally use small lamps, which do not remove darkness from the room excessively. Most of the candles available on the market are to be had at a rate ranging from 1 euro to 10 euro, while the smaller lamps are found in stores even for much less than 3 euro.

The lights have to be suffused, preferably warm in shade, to properly stimulate the ying, in addition to guarantee a more openness of the mind. In the meantime, it is higher now not to region stones inside the room, until there may be inadequate energy to get better, considering that they may disturb rest and sleep, whilst plants need to be used best if the room is excessively represented with the aid of the detail of water . In the end, pay attention to the mirrors too: they ought to never be reflected with each different and, once more, observing the surface, you'll not have a glimpse of the door.

Game of reflexes
Leave the embarrassment out of the bedroom and dare with a

large mirror positioned in front of the bed: not only will it make the room seem suddenly, but it will be a great way to warm the atmosphere in a game of see-not-see decidedly spicy.

Scent of romance

Finally, do not forget an excellent fragrance for your room. Light but intoxicating, it will have to redeem the fresh and clean space, if it then awakens the senses ... What more could you want? the scent of your room or your "intimate" environment must be warm, comfortable and sensual. You can choose between fragrance differences and different aroma diffusion systems for your room. We recommend stick diffusers or water-soluble fragrances that need an electric fragrance diffuser. Choose the right perfume ... it will be the one that will make you remember you for a long time!

Dinner in bed

If having dinner in bed is typically banned from etiquette, making a small exception for an erotic night is possible. You need to avoid serving sweets, too many carbohydrates or meals that crush your stomach, even as fish which include oysters, ginseng and ginger liquids, almonds and cocoa are perfect. Dinner can without problems be completed with a delicious champagne, to be sipped slowly together to increase the erotic price of the meal. Relying on the dishes you have chosen, you need to spend among € 20 and € 80 to put together a full dinner.

Sexy underwear

And because you can not listen totally at the design of the room you certainly have to deliver yourself a moment to buy and wear attractive underwear that stimulates the creativeness of your boyfriend. Do studies and try to discover where you companion's possibilities are orientated: he may love materials consisting of lace, suede, lycra; succinct or extra sober linen vibrant hues that transmit aggression or calm or protection Inside the predominant lingerie stores, the fee of underwear levels from € 20 to € 120.

The right temperature

Whether you choose to give your partner a night of summer or winter fire, it is good to opt for a room with a mild climate which does not spoil the other efforts made due to too hot or too cold. Get fans, which can help the atmosphere become ever sexier, or small stoves to be soberly hidden. The important thing is that the bed cover is also comfortable, neither cold nor stuffy, because these small details must not compromise the romantic evening.

Bathtub

The hot evening can be completed with a nice bath together: here you can indulge yourself with the decorations, adding candles (see above), white enveloping tablecloths, stabilized rose petals, rugs, fragrances and essence diffusers. The water can be enriched with chocolate or milk, to make your bodies smooth and very exciting to the touch. If you are lucky enough to have a bathtub inside the bedroom, it will be even easier to switch from your love bed to the warmth of the water.

Chapter 7. The hottest erogenous zones

The first crucial consideration is that even though the erogenous zones are quite similar for anybody, they are able to range significantly from person to character; in truth they can be greater or much less widespread, greater or less touchy and in a different way disbursed. There are folks who revel in the strongest sensations if they're touched at the lips, others on the breast, others directly at the genital areas.

Sexuality and erogenous zones are topics that aren't typically discussed.

The clinical network has investigated the position - that's pretty intuitive - of those specific and touchy regions of the frame, learning now not most effective the mechanisms that underlie their stimulus, but additionally the effects that the latter have at the brain. Earlier than intending with a extra exact dialogue, it is honestly suitable to recommend a definition of the term.

An erogenous zone is an area of the body whose stimulation, caused by external factors, causes pleasure and excitement. The word "erogeno", which comes from the Greek "eros", means precisely "that generates eros", or "desire" or "love", depending on the context. It is good to specify, to avoid misunderstandings, that these parts that provoke sexual desire are not necessarily located near the genital organs. Another very important aspect to consider is that, contrary to what can be expected on the basis of the knowledge of the anatomical differences between men and women, the erogenous zones are mainly the same for both sexes. The erogenous zones can be divided into three categories: primary, secondary and tertiary.

Tantric sex, also called "the no way" is based on the present moment and the maximum concentration. In order to practice it, the muscles surrounding the sexual organs, the pubic-coccygeal (PC), must function properly.
Specifically, these are three areas:

- the area around the anus.
- the area of the perineum, between the anus and sex.
- the area surrounding sex.

First of all, it is necessary to identify the erogenous zones of the partner, which can vary from person to person. They are divided into three categories: primary, secondary and tertiary. The primary erogenous zones are the lips, the tongue, the breasts and those located in the genital area: the penis and testicles for men, the vulva, the clitoris and the vagina for women.

The secondary erogenous zones are the inner thigh, the buttocks, the neck, the navel, the belly. The tertiary erogenous zones are the palms of the hands, the sole of the foot, the fingers, the back etc.

The body is a mine of sensitive areas to be explored to experience pleasure or strong emotions while making love or just for fun. It really is the wonderland: full as it is of nerve endings capable of sending messages to the brain, the body offers many enjoyable possibilities to experience orgasm or even just very strong sensations (and emotions). And when you are already in "sex mode", it may be enough for your partner to touch certain particularly sensitive areas with your fingers to trigger an earthquake in your lower abdomen. Here is a map of the most sensitive areas of your body.

Men erogenous areas

Male erogenous zones are particularly concentrated around the genital vicinity. As highlighted in professor Turnbull's take a look at, the penis is the primary erogenous region. However, the genital organ of guy is certainly not simple, and is composed of numerous elements which, relying at the case, may be more or less touchy to external stimulations. On this feel, the glans penis represents a question mark for people: whilst, in truth, for a few individuals it's a supply of high-quality delight and sexual preference, for others its stimulation can even be annoying and beside the point.

In people who have now not gone through circumcision, even the typical phimotic ring of the foreskin can be considered as an important erogenous zones: many studies, in fact, confirm that the flap of skin that covers the glans and that can be more or less often it is very rich in nerve endings that cause pleasure to the individual.

Another important erogenous zone present in the area but with which not all men are equipped is the frenulum: this very thin flap of skin that connects the glans and foreskin, in fact, has a significant flow of blood when the penis is erect, and it can be a source of much pleasure if properly stimulated. Further, a moderate stimulation of the scrotum may have superb results earlier than sexual act, even though some guys have hypersensitive reaction to this type of provocation and can be annoyed by it rather than increased libido.

Far from the genital area, the nipples can also be included among the erogenous zones of men, in a similar way to what happens to women; however, the stimulation of the male nipples causes on average less pleasure than in women (in Professo Turnbull's study the men indicated an average intensity relativ to the zone of 4.9 on a scale ranging from 0 to 10).

The perineum and the inner thigh also obtained a very hig score, and it is interesting to underline how the role o stimulation of the head and hair is relevant, with about a poin of difference (in negative) compared to the nipples.

In males, moreover, the stimulation of the ears is surprisingl more exciting than that of the chest. And another interestin fact, in contrast to the latest "fashions", is the very low intensit following the stimulation of the feet: this part of the bod considered by many - at least visually - very erotic, canno therefore be included among the erogenous zones in the 'man.

Women erogenous zones

What are the female erogenous zones? The touching of girl bod parts susceptible to sensory stimulation is, in a few ways, greate complex than that of guy, due to the several areas rich in nerv endings that aren't right away visible.

For example, one of the most exciting and susceptible parts t stimulation, delicate but prolonged, are the internal walls of th vagina. Anatomically, these walls have a layered structure and are equipped with a protective mucosa, but above all they are characterized by a large influx of blood and lymphatic vessels. Just the large spraying that affects the area, and the associated nerve endings, make it very sensitive to touch.

However, it is important to emphasize the extremely high importance of the clitoris. It is not only experience that confirms it, but also data from the scientific literature: the clitoris has a key role in the phenomenon of excitement. From the data reported by Professor Turnbull's study, in fact, it is clear that this organ is by far the most important of the woman's erogenous zones, with a deviation of about 1 point with respect to the inside of the vagina.

Breasts and nipples play the same role with regard to the generation of desire. As regards the nipple, however, it is good to specify that a more important role is played by the areola than the actual breast.

Furthermore, in women, the head and hair can be classified as an "average erogenous" zone: the intensity relative to their stimulation is on average three points lower than the nipples (as opposed to what happened with men), even if between individuals can be very sensitive differences.

Furthermore, in both men and women, the lips are among the strongest erogenous zones: this part of the body very far from the genitals and continuously exposed to the external environment has a different composition than the rest of the epidermis, and is rich in nerve endings that are related to the activation of brain mechanisms that increase libido.

However, even in this case, the differences between individuals can be decisive in defining whether or not the lips are an erogenous zone, contrary to what happens, for example, for the vagina or clitoris. Then there are erogenous zones that seem to be rather overrated. Among these it is possible to count:

The hands, which in some women can provoke a sexual response but which on average do not have a noticeable effect as you can imagine; the hips, which despite being very close to the sexual organs and recognized in the collective imagination as synonymous with femininity, do not have sufficient nerve endings; the feet, for which the same argument applies to men.

In conclusion, it is good to remember that for all these parts of the body, both for women and for men, we speak of trends and averages: the reality of each individual can deviate significantly from mere statistical data. For this reason, it is advisable that all men and women who want to know their body better undergo a real "body mapping". Only with direct experience, in fact, it is possible to determine which parts of one's body generate the greatest stimulus.

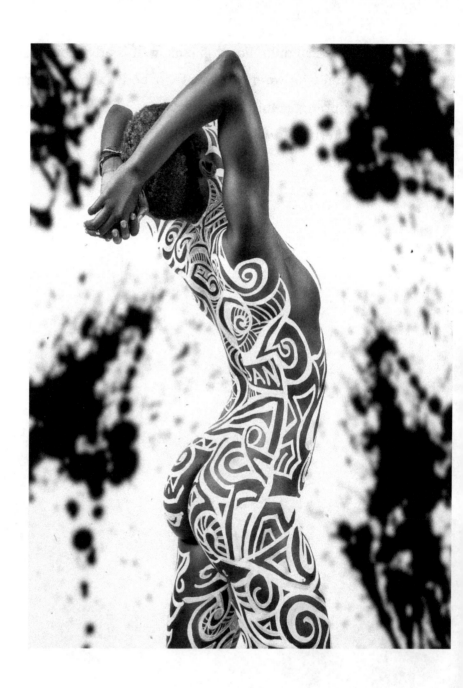

Chapter 8. The Art of Tantric massage

Tantra massage is an art that has an ancient, or even millenary, origin. This massage technique has always been surrounded by an aura of mystery and history, of specific movements and techniques that have the power to soothe the spirit, to improve sexuality and the psychological state. It is a global experience that produces sensory pleasure by improving self-perception through the stimulation of the body's energy points.

Tantric massage is an ancient Indian practice which, through light and circular touches, stimulates the knowledge of oneself, of the other and leads to a state of well-being that is at the same time union and liberation: let's see all the advantages.

Although tantric massage has more than five thousand years of existence, many still know little about it. Its primary function, of course, is to arouse or release sensuality, but not necessarily having to do with sex.

Through the tantric massage and the stimulation of certain energetic points of the body, the person who receives it experiences a great sensorial pleasure and at the same time an improvement of the perception of oneself and of one's own awareness. It is a good massage for those who want to increase and increase the knowledge and harmony of the couple.

The same massage technique has the principle of awakening our vital energy, acting on the emotional field and, consequently leading us to pleasure. It all starts with bodily stimuli that aim to achieve orgasmic energy. This reasoning, in fact, closes the almost general maxim that we can only have orgasm in certain positions.

It is not a simple erotic massage - as many think - but a ritual in which all parts of the body are explored and stimulated. The legs, back, feet, arms, legs, reproductive organs, neck, head and face are - in fact - touched with light pressure which relaxes and helps breathing. This particular technique comes from the East and has the aim of making you find harmony and excitement of the senses. You understood well! Tantra massage is - for this reason - very suitable for couples, since it stimulates self awareness - both for those who practice it and for those who receive it. The couple tantra massage is described as a spiritual ritual that connects the mutual desires and emotions of the two people involved.

If you do this massage in pairs, those who perform the massage give all their love to those who receive it. In the same way, the recipient completely abandons himself in the hands of the executor and prepares himself in a state of total trust. Really recommended for those who want to try a rapprochement with their partner in a time of strong stress or couple problems - especially sexual. By having a couple tantra massage, you have the opportunity to discover something new about him. The approach takes place - in fact - both from a sexual and sensory point of view. So let's see what is specifically and how this type of massage is done. Even the ultimate goal of sexual intercourse that derives from tantric massage is not orgasm, where the feelings of both partners are privileged, letting fly to the maximum peaks desires and fantasies. In this way, the couple discovers deeper and more rewarding ways of being together.

As for the methods of execution, two partners who know tantra techniques can massage each other. Alternatively, the couple can go to specialized operators: the masseur will treat the woman, while the masseuse will follow the man; both partners are completely naked. There are also centers where only one masseur takes care of the couple, who for their part is called upon to collaborate in the tantra massage.

Tantra massage can be done with the aid of a expert, as we said, or in a do-it-yourself model. Inside the latter case, care must be taken now not to be too centered on how the recipient is touched and how desirable he is at massaging. We ought to permit ourselves be carried away by sensations and human nature and it ought to all be very instinctive and natural. There will usually be contact among the two all through the entire time: the recipient will be in a position, certainly, to the touch the masseur along with his hand and caress his forms. similarly, the location performs a genuinely critical characteristic, let's have a look at how it have to be.

The tantric couple massage has goals to make everybody better recognised to each of the two people, with particular interest to sexual wants to assist them get to awareness solely throughout sexual intercourse, avoiding to digress with the thoughts. While we've got found out to listen to ourselves, we can also realize the way to listen to the other, as a result building a deeper dating. It appears that thanks to the tantric couple massage, sexual issues which includes untimely ejaculation or impotence for guys, or anorgasmia and shortage of choice in ladies can also be solved, furnished that those issues do no longer have a bodily purpose but are related to stress and moments specifically sensitive of lifestyles.

Before trying out your partner, self-knowledge is critical. Start by list which frame sensations your body likes and aren't necessarily associated with your intercourse or erogenous zones. For women who have issue attaining orgasm, this self-cognizance observation can function like a therapy, broadening the belief of your body and figuring out others who may be preventing you from reaching your pleasure.

The tantric massage down ritual takes location in 3 levels. Inside the first phase, immersed in an environment of indian track, perfumes and tender lights, we devote ourselves to an active harmonization thru meditation: respiration physical games and mantra songs comply with each different. You've got the opportunity to immerse yourself together with your thoughts and listening to in a entire surroundings of peace, that is created through indian tune. Similarly, the alternative senses also wake up and relax, which include the smell with candles and incense, and the sight with using gentle lighting or with chromotherapy. These kind of tools are the manner to start meditation.

Inside the second phase we continue to massage the face and body. The touches are sweet, huge and gradual and are performed along the chakras and nadis or channels where the vital energy passes. The end result is a sensation of massive delight and well-being.

The closing phase is dedicated to rest. Via sipping a natural tea, the enjoy skilled with the operator is shared verbally. The final effect of tantric massage is commonly the notion of a sense of liberation, stability and peace. Just what you need.

The person receiving the massage must free the mind and be present with the body and soul connected at the moment. In this way, you have the opportunity to concentrate on your breathing and - by letting yourself be massaged - get in touch with the other person and with your deepest self. The performer's hand never detaches from the recipient.

There is constant physical contact that ends only at the end of the massage. The movements are not predetermined but characterized by a continuous and harmonious flow of concentric gestures. The person who massages draws the body of the person who receives it with his palm and fingers. Everything is marked by the breath, the caresses and the contact between the two bodies. You can also do it on your bed at home using essential oil - such as coconut oil. The perfect environment is warm and welcoming. Scented candles and soothing music will do the rest.

First, select a massage oil that causes sensuality. From aromatherapy stores to intercourse stores, find an aroma that appeals to both.

Play to stimulate and excite your partner as you typically do, but relying on all of the senses: the sight, stripping you steadily and seductively; touch, letting it caress your body and caress it in flip; the taste, with the flavor of kisses; the experience of scent with the scent of your lover's pores and skin and yours and eventually with listening to, thanks to a whole series of words and expressions of the erotic vocabulary which you understand.

Before starting a tantric massage, it is important to know all the touchy points of your partner's genitals, as well as the whole penis. Stimulate the pleasure potential that can be received by way of stimulating the testicles, massaging the scrotum and stimulating the perineum, all extremely vital regions for sporting out this massage.

Lubrication is crucial for tantric and penis massage. Use mild oil which includes almond oil, that is an ideal moisturizer in an effort to supply more delicacy on your actions making the revel in a sequence of awesome sensations for him.

With his partner lying on his stomach, massage his body from the feet to the nape. Stimulates the most sensitive and erogenous zones. Groin, nadiga, thighs and ears apply.
Be aware of the intensity of the movement. The ideal is that they are both strong and light, made with your fingertips.

Don't forget any area: back, hands, feet, sides of the body ... everything matters!
Ask to be massaged too. Harmony between the couple is very important to obtain the benefits of the practice
Looking deeply into the eyes when possible is also an excellent stimulus.

You will have to use both hands, the movements will be ascending and also descending but in a more delicate way. One of your hands will massage the testicles, the scrotum and the perineum, while the other will dedicate itself to the penis from the base of the shaft to the glans, always maintaining the rhythm and using the hands in their entirety. You have to take the penis and testicles with the whole palm, gently so as not to hurt, but firmly at the same time in order to generate pleasure.

To do a tantric massage, it is important that you yourself let yourself go with pleasure in doing the tantric massage and infuse energy that your partner will immediately perceive. Try to be creative too, let the sexual energy pervade you so that your partner can also enjoy it. Don't limit yourself, don't think if you're doing it right or wrong, take advantage of this practice to increase intimacy and create new complicity.

The advantages of tantra are many, these in fact allow to improve both the emotional and the psycho-physical sphere. Tantric massage allows you to reactivate sexual or repressed energy, you can also enhance your mental well-being and the way you perceive yourself. Finally, it is possible to eliminate stress and recharge one's energies.

Chapter 9. Erotic massage: Lingam and Yoni to reach ecstasy of pleasure

Massage is one of the most intense forms of communication for both mankind and the animal kingdom: even the majority of animal species engages in a seduction ritual that involves the gentle rubbing of bodies.

Lingam massage for him

Lingam massage is a tantric derivation treatment that acts by stimulating the male genital area in order to expand the sensations connected to it, improving its sensitivity, leading to greater awareness of one's emotions and to a stronger psychophysical roots. The lingam massage is a tantric massage exclusively for men, while yoni is for women. The aim is absolutely not to achieve sexual pleasure.

Lingam massage passes through the explosive nature of pleasure which, in our daily life, remains channeled in our intimate, without the possibility of going out, precluded by the possibility of interacting with the energy flows of the body, as it should do in nature.

These impediments give rise to blocks, blocks of energy which then, when invested with emotions, become emotional blocks. The first big benefit is a couple benefit: intimacy never experienced before can be achieved, especially if this massage helps to overcome certain inhibitions in bed - both for men and for women. Another big benefit is that the stimulation of the prostate is healthy in humans. And man can also receive a greater awareness of his own body, just as woman can learn to know all her erogenous zones better. It is better to do everything with your eyes closed, mutual knowledge also has to do with tactile sensations.

In order for the Lingam massage to produce all its benefits, it is essential that it be performed in the most correct and ideal way possible. In the meantime, it is worth preparing the place where the massage will take place. It must be neither too hot nor too cold. It must present a comfortable plan, because the man must lie down and be naked.

Have him lie on his back after putting a pillow under his head and one under his pelvis. Her legs must be slightly spread apart and bent in a relaxed way. As if she were getting into a panties to make the family jewels take air. In lingam massages there is nothing rude and friction is not foreseen: get an erotic massage oil and sprinkle your hands and genitals. Everything will be more pleasant for him and for you it will be easier to perform fluid and linear movements.

Relaxation is the basis of everything

It's far essential that the donor and recipient are absolutely at ease, ready with goodwill, not prosthesis so one can obtain well-being, because to be able to come by means of itself, in a totally natural manner. throughout the lingam rub down, the electricity between guy and woman should go with the flow freely so that the energies can come into ideal concord, synchronize and harmonize synergistically and rhythmically.

Lingam massage works via focusing on disposing of the emotional, physical and mental blockages caused by an accumulation of pollutants and when these are eliminated, bodily, emotional and religious fitness is substantially advanced. All in a synchronic way.

This is because, always through the Lingam massage, the energy, the life force, what is precisely called "Prana", is able to flow around and through the body, inside and outside it, embracing all the spheres of the 360 degrees our existence.

In order for this to take place, it is important to perform the massage in the best way possible, therefore it is essential to approach a fully relaxed body and state of mind.

How breathing should be

Lingam massage should be performed in a calm and pleasant environment, with a comfortable, preferably warm temperature. It would be ideal to opt for soft lighting with scented candles, sweet melodies in the background in order to create a sensual atmosphere. To begin the massage, both partners must sit or stand in contact with their hands or look into each other's eyes. Breathing should be synchronized starting with deep breaths that fill the lungs.

It is important to make sure that during the Lingam massage the breathing remains deep for both the donor and the recipient, so that the connection of the hearts remains and the energy continues flowing. The energy of the senses is, in fact, a powerful force but if suffocated it can really hurt the soul, as well as the body.

Well, when harnessed, this energy can induce high levels of emotional, physical and sensual pleasure, because it is our very nature that re-emerges in all its entirety and its fullness. This is the keystone, this is the reason why Lingam massage promises so many benefits. The pressure to be exercised must be right and must take place on the muscles alternately between stroking and kneading.

As you massage, apply light pressure to slow down any tension by pressing forward and releasing back slightly and gently at the end of each movement.

Muscle stimulation must be carried out through a series of particular ordered and delicate movements which gently relax the muscles involved. The affected body part can be massaged by following three maneuvers:

Touching: it consists of very energetic, but very delicate maneuvers designed to ensure a relaxing effect as if it were stroking. These should be performed with slow circular movements. This effect calms the nervous system;

Kneading: it is performed with maneuvers that act on the muscle and connective tissue and with pressure always accompanied by circular movements of the fingers;

Clutch: this maneuver requires greater pressure as it is aimed at mobilizing the tissues of the area by improving blood circulation. In truth, these maneuvers should be carried out critically, following certain steps, choosing - obviously not randomly - when to perform one and when the other, also with full and exact knowledge of the precise times required for each step.

The woman does not have to, but it is certainly better for a number of reasons: it reinforces intimacy and maybe she is even more comfortable. It begins with stroking the whole body: the head, legs, abdomen, arms and so on. It does not come immediately to the highlight.

The penis is the big protagonist, but you have to awaken it little by little. You can start by massaging the inner part of the thighs, then moving to the groin and pubis. Make slow, soft movements and adjust by observing his reactions. Approach the testicles and caress them with circular movements and cupped hands. Ask him if he wants more pressure: not all men like to be crushed, but some do.

Then we move on to the actual penis massage, extending also on the testicles, on the perineum and finally on the prostate. During all the steps, you have to breathe deeply: never hold your breath, relaxation is a must. Massage the lingam alternating different movements and rhythms: go up and down with your hands, perform rotational movements on the rod, dedicate yourself to the base and then go up to the glans and vice versa.

Thanks to the atmosphere and the celestial vision of you fumbling down there, the orgasm of your him may not be long in coming. Pay attention to the rhythm of his breathing and his movements and, when you notice that he is about to come, slow down and go back to other areas. These are the first steps for him to learn editing, a technique that could be very useful between the sheets.

More sacred than the penis there is only the P point, or the prostate. Stimulate it from the outside by massaging the perineum, or the area between the testicles and anus, with your fingertips and knuckles. Then, only if he agrees, insert a finger (or a prostate vibrator) into the anus and try to reach the prostate, a walnut-shaped gland. Massage it gently and with circular movements.

Some men have prejudices about approaching the prostate, so one must be extremely delicate and not make the man feel raped. In fact, it is good to let him know first what lingam massage consists of, because you risk getting to this point and losing all the intimacy gained until then. We must always remember that we are talking about a massage, not a prostate exam (although maybe it can be useful to understand if everything is going well in those parts). The massage cannot be stopped, or damage is done to the body, which, according to tantra, is releasing its energies.

And then relax!

Decide collectively if you want the lingam massage to give up with sexual intercourse or a liberating orgasm on your hands. Anyways, at the end of the erotic massage, relax each, taking time to dedicate yourself to the sensations of your body and to percentage the experience you have lived.

Understand that lingam can't be improvised on a technical degree. If a easy neck massage can be finished with a little guide skill and imagination, the identical cannot be carried out with lingam. The strength will build, disperse and spread over the complete body and sooner or later our could be able to enjoy strong, all-natural pleasure.

The Yoni massage for her
The female counterpart of the lingam massage is the yoni massage: "yoni" has a Sanskrit origin and means "vagina" or in any case refers to the female sexual organ. It is in all respects similar: it is not a simple masturbation, it is the son of tantra and therefore allows the development of energy and a great

intimacy among those who practice it. When you get to the pelvis, you begin to intensively massage the clitoris - taking care not to reach orgasm, even if in the end ... it can happen - and then move on to the search for the G-spot and the stimulation of other afferent erogenous zones. If your partner is a woman even better: at the end of the massage you can exchange parts.

Some refer to the woman's vagina as a "sacred temple". This is because the vagina is a very erogenous zone and deserves to be exploited in different ways, overcoming the spheres of oral sex and simple penetration. In the Tantra philosophy, Yoni is considered with respect and love for followers.

The main goal of the Yoni massage is to make the woman deeply relax and experience sensations that she has never experienced in her entire life. In addition, the massage performed by men's fingers further extends the degree of intimacy between the couple, therefore essential for the health of the relationship. The partner of the massage is called "donor", to give the woman all the pleasure she deserves and should never expect anything in return.

Know that to do the Yoni massage in your partner you have to be selfless, you should never do the massage - which can also generate multiple orgasms in the woman - expect something in return or a pleasure. Sex after the massage can also happen, but usually this is not the rule, especially if the woman enjoys and is already exhausted with so much pleasure.

Although this is not a sexual technique for men, it can be very pleasant for him, since he can see his partner up close as he has never seen before, trembling with so much heat and moaning like crazy. Which man has never thought of leaving a woman in this state, even with her powerful fingers? So learn the Yoni massage technique and apply your loved one!

Prepare the environment
Before you start, you must be careful to prepare the environment. In tantra, the place where sexual activities are given is very important, because it directly affects each person's entire process and mental state. Putting a half light on the environment, smelling incense, flowers, lighting candles, arranging curtains, scarves and colored cushions can create a totally favorable atmosphere for what will come next.

Remember to put a silent ambient sound to balance the space. Human beings are sensitive to the senses, therefore the activation of the sense of smell, hearing, sight and even touch can allow the experience to be more intense for the woman and increase her interaction with her. Even as a donor you will fee more relaxed in developing the technique.

First a nice shower

One of the recommendations of the Yoni massage is to take a relaxing shower before proceeding step by step. The woman can bathe alone by simply lathering her or throwing water or you can participate in the bathroom by starting the ritual of connection and intimacy between you. Try to make this moment something special, without haste and try to enjoy each other' presence. This bath will bring more vigor to both, as well as disinfect the entire region you will explore.

Balanced breathing

For Yoni massage to work, it is important that your breathing is synchronized. Hence, man and woman should seek balance of breathing, a calm, regular and calm breath. Shortness of breath shows insecurity, anxiety or even excitement in advance and the Yoni massage indicates that hormones are controlled and the woman is completely relaxed, available and confident with everything she will feel soon. Inhale and exhale together until you are in perfect harmony, if necessary you can also do a yoga session before finding the balance you need.

Disconnect from the entirety

You and your accomplice should be completely involved with each different and with the space you've organized for the interest. Consequently, it is recommended to forget about the entirety out of doors of that area all worldly and material things. Turn off the smartphone, notebook, if they have children worry about having anyone at home during the day, if they have dog or other pet, they leave in another room, close the door, unplug the intercom, the phone, close the windows, the curtains and then immerse yourself in the universe you created. Glaringly now not best material matters are critical, however you two ought to also make an effort not to disperse concentration with thoughts about problems and other concerns from outside.

Placement

Make sure to make the woman comfortable. You can place it on the cushions and leave it upside down so you can observe the massage, the movements you perform and even your image, to make it even more stimulated. He may want to keep his eyes closed so that he can feel all the vibrations more fully, it will depend on the choice of each.

Put a pillow covered with a towel on your hips. The legs should be separated and the knees bent in the typical position of that woman when she is about to give birth. Her genital organ must be fully exposed to you as a donor, who can sit in front of her to be able to perform all movements with ease and free access.

Start of touches

Start by massaging your legs, thighs, breasts, abdomen and other regions before reaching the vagina. Pour a small amount of lubricant, which can be purchased in specialty stores and sex shops. Then squeeze the outer lip between your thumb and forefinger and slide up and down with slow and precise movements.

Then, do the same movement on the inner lip, always calmly, making the woman accustomed to her touch. It is recommended that the couple maintain eye contact during the massage to intensify the sensation and exchange between the two.

Since the preference for intensity, speed and pressure varies from woman to woman, the recipient should tell the donor how she prefers while experiencing the sensations.

This will make it easier for you to find the right spot for his pleasure. But it limits the conversation, since prolonged speech can be a factor in dispersing the massage.

Focus on the clitoris

The clitoris is a complex structure, similar to the glans penis in the male sex. So it is extremely sensitive and erogenous, it can be up to four times more sensitive than the glans penis, in fact. This is because it has between 6 and 8 thousand nerve endings, which contributes to being one of the largest female pleasure generators.

When massaging the clitoris, it is necessary to make circular movements clockwise and counterclockwise. Slowly insert the middle finger of your right hand into the vagina and make various movements - using your right hand has everything to do with the polarity of Tantra, then follow the instructions.

G-spot or "Holy Place"

Massage the inside of the vagina with your finger, varying the speed, depth and pressure. With your finger still inside the vagina, do the "come here" movement over and over again. In this area you will be in contact with a spongy tissue that is located under the public bone and behind the clitoris. Remember that the G-spot has much less sensitivity than the clitoris, so you can be much more energetic: the best way to stimulate it is to bend your fingers towards the palm of your hand, as if you were saying to a person 'come here'.

When you feel that your woman is very close to orgasm, the best thing you can do is keep pressing it but without moving. The simple pressure should bring her to orgasm and if not, don't worry. The purpose of the yoni massage is to bring the woman back into contact with her sexual energy; if you have dedicated yourself to his yoni with attention and love, surely you have succeeded. Otherwise we will have to start over and we bet that your partner will be more than happy.

Finalization

At the same time you can use the little finger of the right hand to insert it into the woman's anus, obviously if she accepts. So, you can extend his feeling of pleasure with the Yoni massage. In the meantime, you can use your free hand (left hand) to massage the breast, abdomen or clitoris. The woman, completely sensitive to touch, can even cry with sensations or start. If what tantra adepts call 'side effect', or orgasm, should occur, we suggest that you do not stop immediately but try to continue to gently stimulate the yoni, perhaps in the area of the clitoris with the palm of your hand open always reminding the woman to continue breathing deeply. And you might even get her multiple orgasms.

Chapter 10. Top essential oils to use for Tantra massage

In tantra, essential aphrodisiac oils are used to stimulate and modulate desire, to release and eliminate tension. The instinctive and emotional side and is able to significantly influence the reactions of the autonomous system which is directly related to pleasure and sexual reactions.

An example is the subconscious perception of another person's natural scent, a component that convincingly influences a partner's choice. This mechanism, which has been widely studied in animal behavior, is related to mating and reproduction processes and plays an important role. Also in humans. It is no coincidence that strong physical attraction is often determined and conveyed by smell. Many sexual abnormalities or relationship difficulties can be attributed to an entirely instinctive rejection of another person's scent, which is unpleasant, disturbing and thus leads to progressive elimination. This is why essential oils can help us overcome certain sexual disorders.

Aphrodisiac essential oils: perfume and seduction

The relationship between the art of seduction and perfume has many ancient roots, as does the concept of aphrodisiac perfume.

This is a relative term, not an absolute term: everyone recognizes themselves in a particular scent and not in others because of their own experiences and temperaments and therefore finds an essence that pleases them than others.

Decisions and smell sense preferences can also change in the course of life, and individual reactions develop constantly and vary depending on experience, needs, desire for stability or desire to change. This attention makes us realize that there is no perfume for anyone who can be tempted and inclined for pleasure. However, there are some essential oils which, because of their specific aroma, can fall into a vital dimension of human experience, sexuality, more than others.

Aphrodisiac essential oils: how to use them
It can be very useful to practice massage with essential oils, such as coconut oil, cinnamon oil, lavender oil, basil oil, etc. These oils, in addition to promoting the sliding of the hands on the recipient's body, will flood the room with a pleasant fragrance.

- *Personal perfumes:* They can be used as real perfumes if diluted in alcohol.

- *Massage creams and oils:* to customize neutral creams

and vegetable oils to be applied on the face or body for massage with essential oils or simply to perfume your moisturizing and nourishing lotion.

- *Stimulating bath:* 10 drops in the water of the bathtub, before your performance under the sheets, will help stimulate your desire and prepare for intercourse.

- *Environmental diffusion:* 1gc for each square meter of the environment, by air diffusion with an essence burner or in the humidifiers of the radiators.

Essential oils for her

- *Ylang-ylang essential oil:* helps to awaken the senses, in case of frigidity and impotence, and for those who cannot let go; removes doubt, insecurities and blocked feelings. It is of great help in repressed femininity because it releases joy, sensuality, euphoria and internal security. It creates harmony in case of contrasts, anger, resentment and frustration, because it promotes understanding and forgiveness, dissolves disappointments and offenses and restores the desire to love.

- *Rose essential oil:* opens and strengthens the heart relaxes the soul and activates the disposition for tenderness and love, because it develops patience devotion and self-esteem. It gives joy and dispels negative thoughts, balancing negative emotions caused by anger jealousy and stress

- *Patchouli essential oil:* induces the pituitary gland to produce endorphin (euphoric) useful for those who cannot let go (frigidity) or have a drop in libido: increases concentration and energy. Recommended for older people who, because of their social and professional life, have to control their physical impulses, and suffer from psycho-physical exhaustion or sexual disorders.

Essential oils for him

- *Pine essential oil:* it is linked to the male universe, it helps those who have difficulty getting in touch with their virility and expressing it. It has a stimulating action, useful in the treatment of impotence, frigidity, in case of decreased libido.

- *Ginger essential oil:* it has a strong action (i.e. it

determines the recall of blood in the most superficial layers of the skin, heating the area and lightening the inflammation to the underlying layers thanks to the subtraction of blood). Ginger essential oil gives warmth to the body and helps awaken and warm the dormant senses.

- *Sandalwood essential oil:* works by balancing sexuality with the spirit, promoting the integration of the sacred with the profane: for this reason it is used in tantra yoga schools to transform sexual energies into spiritual energies. It is therefore not a direct aphrodisiac, as its action is mainly meditative and directed towards the interior: it is rather aimed at subjects who experience the sexual topic with superficiality. Transform sexual energy by elevating it on the spiritual level. It reduces aggression and violent instincts, eases exasperation, and releases blocked sexual energy.

Chapter 11. The best tantric sex positions

Tantra's position make possible to enhance harmony and balance in partner relationships and, above all to rediscover sexuality that is almost satisfying, almost spiritual. The Tantra positions refers to a refined oriental philosophy which involves reversing the traditional roles of men/women. The active part is the woman and has a duty to transfer her "cold energy" to men who convert it to "heat energy". In this phase you don't want to reach orgasm, you want to increase your vitality.

Tantra positions can help us explore the sexual pleasure that our bodies can experience with greater satisfaction. Therefore, it is not only possible to increase orgasm, but also the quality of erotic intimacy. In one of the metaphors used by tantra, the body is like a drum. The joy we feel depends not so much on our partner, but on ourselves: the more we know each other and realize who we are and our bodies, the stronger our voice and intense joy.

Tantric sex is only recommended for people who are very close because it is more mental than physical and shows all the psychological and motivational problems that underlie a relationship. At the same time, this is a practice that struggles regularly and allows you to build deep and passionate relationships, true spiritual enlightenment. To overcome this in the best way, you don't need to be afraid to try something new. Only with an open mind and heart will it be possible to reach full pleasure. You must then decide to spend at least one hour a week on your sexuality, even if you are tired or stressed. Tantric sex is actually able to activate the body and make it stronger and more energetic.

Here a new position can help renew your passion. Before examining the best position of tantric sex, very appropriate and deep foreplay must be followed to achieve complete physical and mental satisfaction. In this case, couple must be in a state of complete relaxation during tantric love.

You have to pay attention and observe each other, look at each other and listen each other. Only when this balance is reached, only when the outflow of glances and maximum inhalation, then and only then can we continue. Tantra does not need to be jumped into a thousand love positions to reach orgasm. Basically four are enough:

Man above:
In this position, the face of the man and the woman are in close

contact, therefore you can look each other in the eyes, kiss eac other passionately, touch and smell, using all 5 senses. Whei man feels he is about to ejaculate, he can stop.

Woman above:

When the woman is in this position, she can direct th penetration in the most sensitive areas of the vagina, i particular towards the point G. In this way she is able to reach multitude of orgasms. The man can stimulate the clitoris witl his hands, or kiss the breast, increasing mutual excitement

One next to the other. "The position of the spoon".

This position requires some coordination of the couple. Man ca penetrate even if he is not in full erection.

Man behind

It is a more carnal and passionate position, but also in this cas the slowness of the movement can extend the pleasure t infinity.

The usual position in tantric sex is a position where a woman sits on her partner's thighs, legs her crossed behind his back and hugs his partner in a warm embrace. This way you can also look into his eyes and build deeper connections. The more sporty, the more support, like weight. Now let's look at the other top 10 sex positions:

1. The first position sees the man lying in a supine position, with the woman lying on top in a complementary way. The latter must keep her hands on the ground and her arms straight, raising slightly at the level of the torso towards her partner.

2. The second position sees the woman sit on the man's legs, crossing their own behind the partner's back. The partners then hold each other tightly in a warm embrace. This is probably the most famous one, typical of tantric sex.

3. The third position is a kind of more complex version of the previous one. It sees the two partners sitting opposite each other, always in a crossed pose. The man with his arms supports the partner's knees at the elbow and vice versa.

4. The fourth position of tantric sex requires the help of a support high enough to allow it to be performed. The partner lies down on the piece of furniture with the pelvis practically at the end of the same. The man, standing, supports the woman's legs on the sole of the foot, keeping them straight.

5. Even the fifth position of tantric sex requires the help of a support such as the armrest of an armchair or sofa. The woman remains seated, keeping her legs apart, with her knees gently bent and her feet firmly on the ground. Instead, the man remains standing and the woman holds him tightly on his shoulders.

6. Preferably on the ground, with the help of a pillow or a comfortable carpet, the man, on his knees, lifts the legs of the beloved who is lying supine in front of him. Keeping the woman's knees bent, the man must approach and support the pelvis, while the woman must leverage her arms and back to support herself. This is the sixth best position of tantric sex.

7. On armchairs and / or sofas it is possible to experiment with an inverted position with respect to those described so far: the man remains seated, possibly with his legs bent and his feet firmly on the ground, while the woman places her legs on the shoulders of the companion while sitting on the pelvis, arching the back.

8. The eighth position of tantric sex is that which sees the partner sitting on his legs, that is, with the buttocks close to the feet. The woman, sitting on the pelvis, turns her back on the

man keeping her knees bent and her feet firmly on the ground, arching her back slightly forward.

9. A variant of the previous described position is that which always sees the woman facing the man. The couple keeps both calves resting on the ground and the rest of the body perpendicular to the floor. They push each other at the pelvis level.

10. The last position of tantric sex involves a singular technique, very effective. It is one that sees the two partners placed in a complementary position, with the right foot and calf resting on the ground, the knee bent and the upper body perpendicular in the calf. To proceed in the position in question you will have to make a kind of lunge with the left leg, bending it forward. The same will be possible for the woman, with inverted limbs in this case.

Positions are chosen according to their preferences: it is about mastering both sexual energy and maximizing pleasure. However, these are just a few suggestions that might benefit those who are starting in this art that combines sex and meditation. Thanks to tantric sex, we become free from boundaries, prejudices, and false beliefs. Sex is part of everything, it is the basis of our existence, but habits can ruin the beauty of these acts of love, which are often done mechanically.

Tantric sex is the key to opening the door to pleasure, releasing sexual energy and allowing you to experience certain feelings during very long periods of sexual intercourse. This oriental discipline changes the approach to sex, which has been rejected as an instrument to harmonize the senses, harmony of partners, inner and outer balance and all undergo unique and very sensory experiences.

Chapter 12. Tantra daily exercises you can do at home

Try to think of the typical sex, without romanticism: it is what you do quickly, with him who often comes before her, few looks and many fixed thoughts. "Will him notice my cellulite?" - "Do I have enough for her?". We are so far away from the concept of tantric sex, of slow and overwhelming spiritual and physical union that we all dream of as teenagers. You may have heard of tantric sex thanks to some stars, but few really know what we are talking about.

It is a real philosophy that reveals how to learn to have sex for hours, how to prolong pleasure indefinitely and how to get to experience an extreme and deep orgasm. Or not to try it completely, discovering a high level of pleasure in which you don't need a sudden peak of sensations (incredible, but true!). If you are looking for a way to turn your sexual experiences as a couple into something supernatural, then in this chapter I explain everything you need to know about tantra for two. And goodbye #forever to poor sex.

Tantra and its techniques are not easy, but neither are they impossible. Be careful: tantric practices are for very close couples. They will prove an epic fail if there is a lack of confidence, feeling and desire at the top. Ready to try? There is no need to buy a guide to tantric sex, just start getting involved with the four basic tantric exercises:

1. **Live the present moment and be aware of your body:** listen to yours and its body, listen to your breaths, look intensely in your eyes, love every detail of each other. There is no room to think about what you need to do next, what commitments you have to make, what problems you have at work, what physical defects your partner might see. During tantric love, love every detail of yourself and the other. No mental limit, no physical limit, no prejudice. Kiss each other, touch each other, observe each other all the time of the relationship.

2. **Rhythm and movement are fundamental:** they are essential to put energy into circulation and must be done in harmony. Partners move together, at the same speed, possibly slowly and deeply, especially at the pelvis level. No fervor in penetration, please. It must be almost a dance.

3. **Tantra breathing is a must:** how to prolong pleasure if not controlling the breath? The more relaxed and soft it

is, the more it oxygenates the erogenous zones. The best would be to synchronize your breath with that of your partner: try to inhale counting to six, hold your breath for six seconds and exhale for another six.

4. **Prolonged coitus:** the sensations are so deep that it will be natural for you to postpone orgasm. It won't have to be your goal, you won't have to chase it, but you won't have to hold it back if you feel it's exploding. The male does not even need a full erection: it is enough that the penis remains inside to stimulate it with contraction of the pelvic muscles and continue to experience super pleasure. It is called a valley orgasm and arises from listening to the sensations: the warmth, the softness of the skin, the perfume, the features of the partner and so on.

Many wonder if tantric sex really works. To be an erotic moment in a partner, it is necessary to follow a series of "tricks". First of all, you must focus on your body and the rhythm of the movement to increase energy circulation. Voice broadcasts may not be blocked or suppressed for any reason. With tantric sex, you must feel free to express your pleasure 100%. Finally, deep breathing also contributes to pleasure. To improve results, there are exercises that must be done with a partner to improve all areas of sexual performance. For example, you can learn to breathe correctly with your diaphragm. You must inhale to six, hold your breath for six seconds, and exhale for six seconds. In addition, women need to understand where the perineal area is located, it can only be used to stimulate orgasm with pelvic muscles without sudden movements.

Observe with one's conscience everything that happens within oneself: thoughts, bodily sensations, mainly breathing, and emotions. It begins by sitting down and observing one's breathing which, prolonged over time, slowly changes and becomes more fluid. And it begins to involve more and more parts of the body. Those who breathe with their chest, for example, begin to feel breathing also in the abdomen and vice versa.

At first it may not be so easy to concentrate on breathing letting go of thoughts and worries. The important thing is to take the first step and be constant. As for bodily sensations, macroscopic details such as the back that pulls or the buttocks on the pillow are felt at first, then gradually we can perceive what the tantrics call a swarm of bees, a subtle vibration throughout the body.

However, this only happens when the body has almost completely released all the tensions.

Having strong sexual muscles is the basis for becoming tantric lovers, otherwise it is impossible to think of controlling them and practicing Tantra successfully. There is a specific group of muscles that surrounds the sexual organs, of extreme importance for general health and for the functioning of the latter. The correct name for these muscles is pubo-coccygeal or "PC muscle", as we usually prefer to call them.

This group of muscles is referred to as a single muscle since it functions as a unit during sexual activity, but in reality it can be divided into three areas:

- the area around the anus;
- the area of the perineum, between the anus and the sex;
- the area surrounding sex.

A strong and trained "PC muscle" is the key to good sexuality for both men and women.

Contractions of the PC muscle
One of the best ways to train and keep strong your "computer

muscles" is through contractions. When you start to contract, you might not be able to divide your PC muscle into three parts, but the entire area will contract. Don't worry, it's normal. With time and commitment, you can understand and practice it separately. Below I show you very effective training which includes two types of contractions.

Short checks. Quickly contract and relax the PC muscle (or part of it) by holding the contraction for 1 second and releasing for 1 second. 10 in a row are performed for each sequence; five sequences are made for each training session that will be done 1 time per day.

Long checks. Contract and relax the PC muscles by holding the contraction for 30 seconds and releasing for 2 seconds. There are 3 consecutive for each sequence. Five sequences are made for each session that will be done 1 time per day.

Below I list other very effective systems to train your sexuality and that of the couple, day by day.

Tantric masturbation. Tantric masturbation does not disturb relationship, on the contrary, it enriches it. Are you coming to practice it? Just like tantric sex. Regulate breathing, focus on the sensations, the looks and the moment you are experiencing. You must feel your sensual and sexual fire exploding in the pelvis area.

The couple Tantra Massage. Not an erotic massage tout court, but a real experience in which all parts of the body are explored and stimulated with light pressures that relax, excite and emotionally connect the two partners. Empty mind, synchronized and regular breathing: focus on each sensation. There is no precise technique: those who massage must use essential oil and caress the other's body with their fingers or the palm of the hand. Duration, pressure and rhythm can apply. Relaxation guaranteed for a preliminary beyond perfection.

The Tantra Kundalini massage. A very specific variant of couple tantra massage is the kundalini tantra massage. It was created to stimulate the first chakra located in the perineum area: partner lying on the belly, it massages the area between the anus and the genitals and goes up along the spine to awaken all the kundalini energy that goes up - chakra after chakra - up to the head. Also essential oil, delicacy and relaxation for overwhelming sensations.

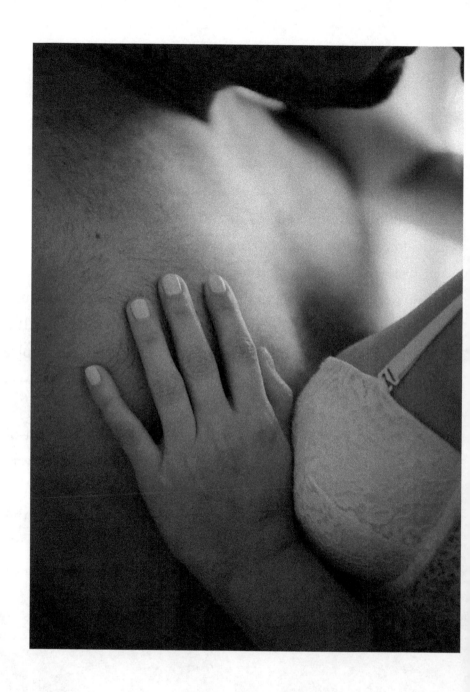

Chapter 13. Eiaculation control: the best remedies and exercises

Unfortunately for some men, orgasm comes too fast. Sometimes almost immediately. Preventing you from enjoying all the sensations of pleasure. And leaving the woman unfulfilled. As is well known, ejaculation is the process by which seminal fluid is expelled externally through the urethra. There is talk of premature ejaculation when the man does not control the coming of the orgasm, which happens suddenly, without the ability to manage the seminal fluid. In fact, reaching orgasm quickly in particular situations is an absolutely normal thing. However, if this happens systematically, with any partner and in any condition, it is a disorder that needs to be addressed.

In 10 percent of cases of premature ejaculation, man reaches orgasm during the foreplay phase; much more often, that is, in the remaining 90 percent of cases, it manages to sustain the preliminaries, even if they last for a long time, but it is unable to control ejaculation when the moment of penetration comes.

During the ejaculation, as in erective mechanism, the pelvic floor muscles are therefore involved. The rhythmic movement of the pelvis, which leads to orgasm, is in fact of a contractual type. At this stage, muscle tension - at the level of the penis but also of nearby muscles - increases dramatically.

Ejaculation, although lasting only a few seconds, is not a single process, as you have just read, but occurs in two stages. In the first phase, with the contraction of the pelvic muscles, the sperm is pushed out of the testicles and introduced into the vas deferens, connected to the penis. It is collected at the base of the urethra, pending expulsion in the final ejaculatory act.

In the second phase, which occurs at a very short distance, the different bundles of the pelvic muscles, for example the ischiocavernosus and the bulbocavernosus muscles, contract and the seminal fluid, through the urethra, is pushed out. Normally the contraction of the pelvic muscles is an involuntary act. But through the control on the muscles that is obtained thanks to the exercises of pelvic gymnastics, or intimate gymnastics, it is possible to recognize the difference between the two phases and lengthen the response times of the final contraction. And consequently increase the duration of the relationship.

Thus, a good pelvic floor condition allows people to manage the pleasure stage. On the other hand, if the pelvic floor bundles are weak and poorly perceived, this sense of mastery is lacking.

Muscles do not respond to stimuli for contraction and relaxation: it is not possible to control various states of excitement until the final phase. And the connection ends prematurely with premature ejaculation.

The remedies for premature ejaculation involve various spheres: if, in fact, the psychological or relational factors have been identified as causative or maintenance of dysfunction factors, cognitive-behavioral therapy is the treatment of choice. It provides a targeted path aimed at increasing ejaculatory latency times through the development of awareness about the physical sensations that precede orgasm. This goal is achieved both through behavioral techniques such as stop-start, and through cognitive work to manage performance anxiety.

Mastering the stage of sexual pleasure not only helps men solve the problem of premature ejaculation. But also to increase efficiency: Sexual intercourse lasts longer and desires increase. According to various scientific studies, premature ejaculation is a problem that occurs when male cannot recognize the sensation that predisposes to orgasm. In short, a person ejaculates too quickly when he cannot concentrate at the right time when it will need to concentrate to stop the ejaculation reflex.

So, based on this theory, learning pelvic exercises is very useful because, besides strengthening muscles, perception, awareness, and ability to focus when ejaculation increases and learn how to deal with it. Intimate gymnastics exercises make you more aware of your sexual system and gradually gain the ability to control the sensation of orgasm. This is not a new technique. The texts of Tantra and Tao, ancient spiritual disciplines, illustrate this practice. Orgasm - and thus ejaculation - occurs under the direct control of the will. And that can be postponed, delayed, detained, intensified. In short: it is managed.

Men say that intimate gymnastics has enabled them to control their pelvic contractions and control their duration. Targeted exercise increases the sensitivity, coordination and concentration of these muscles. Ejaculation disorders also affect cases where ejaculation is delayed or does not occur.

One of the causes is a hypertonic pelvic floor, i.e. a continuous and constant muscle contraction, which maintains a protracted state of tension, weakening the muscle fibers. Muscle hypertonia makes the pelvis rigid and blocked. And it takes away from the muscle cells their natural contractile ability. The urethral sphincter cannot create the alternation of contraction and relaxation necessary to allow the passage of sperm. And ejaculation is hindered.

Therefore, intimate gymnastics makes sense for all ejaculatory disorders if done correctly. In short, there is almost always pelvic weakness, although there are more than one causes of premature ejaculation. Therefore, contraction of pelvic floor muscles can be very useful in controlling sperm emission in this problem. It can also help to practice progressive relaxation techniques that help you achieve muscle relaxation in a short amount of time. A particular form of relaxation is that of the pelvic musculature. In fact, these muscles facilitate or inhibit ejaculation and it is the same muscles that stop urination. By contracting and releasing them voluntarily during the day (Kegel Exercises) it is possible to reach a degree of awareness that allows you to relax them and delay ejaculation.

Another powerful way to premature ejaculation is to maintain relaxation even during masturbation. So for this purpose, it is necessary to practice autoeroticism by repeatedly gaining and losing erections, by caressing and focusing attention only on physical sensations. Once you are familiar with this procedure, you can introduce a stop-start technique (Semans, 1956).

In this exercise, you will learn how to maintain a high level of arousal without reaching orgasm. During masturbation, the man always tries to reach the maximum level of arousal - around seven on a scale from zero to ten - and then stops stimulation when he has an orgasm. The urgency of ejaculation will subside in a few seconds and at that time the man will continue stimulation. If you repeat this exercise every week, you can increase the time delay and familiarize yourself with the sensations before orgasm.

When men are in a stable relationship, it helps to create a climate of calm and intimacy in couples, for example by openly and respectfully discussing what they like or dislike about the relationship and what causes emotions and emotions. sexual activity. Creating a positive and inviting atmosphere makes it easier to reduce anxiety and strengthen sexual relations and partners.

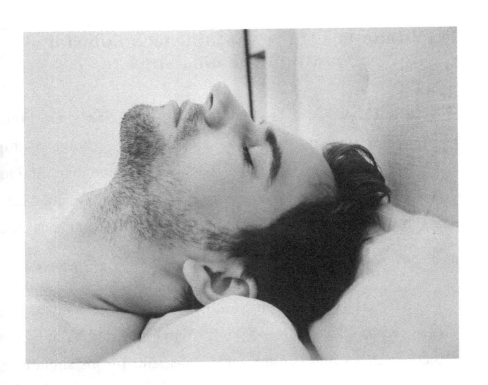

Chapter 14. The shocking technique for a multidimensional orgasm

Have you ever heard of "Valley orgasm"? At first glance, this expression suggests that it is a concept in dichotomy with another: where there is a valley there is also a mountain. And in fact it is like this: "upstream orgasm" and "downstream orgasm" are in fact concepts related to tantric sex, so let's talk about the spiritual side of sex and sexuality.

To understand, let's go behind the figurative image: a mountain, designed as a fixed stereotype, is a large inverted V, in which there is an ascent, a summit and a descent. In this similitude, the ascent is represented by all those actions that are carried out when having sex - from foreplay, to penetration, up to a change of position, etc. When you get to the top of the mountain, you feel the orgasm of the mountain, but the descent is sweet and pleasant, not fast and immediate. The mountain orgasm does not disappear immediately but, if "cultivated" in the right way, it can allow you to reach the valley orgasm.

It is important not to detach after having reached both orgasms: if you don't separate, you can reach the valley orgasm, a state of deep well-being and closeness, love and deep meditation that somehow interpenetrate as the two bodies have penetrated just before. But it is possible only through silent observation, just before returning to normal, to the state that precedes coitus. Afterwards there can also be moments of pampering, indeed they are very important, almost essential, perhaps through massages with oils, good music and a little scented candles.

To reach the Valley orgasm you don't have to do anything. Yes, that may seem absurd, but actually all the actions taken before orgasm are the speculative and meditative phases of the relationship.

But be careful: this does not mean that you have to dress or fall asleep right after the relationship. This is what Tantra recommends to avoid. Sex is a sacred moment and must be treated as such. We then follow the relationship phases to better understand how to behave, to do the best of sex and to have experiences that connect the body and soul.

You are in bed - or wherever you like - with your partner. There are the foreplay and then the actual relationship which may or may not include penetration. The relationship culminates in the Valley Orgasm - when and if it arrives - after which you take your time. Staying close, embraced, in contemplation. The ideal is to reach climax together, but it is something that can come thanks to a deep mutual knowledge and practice - sometimes also of a sentimental nature, not only distinctly sexual. So after the climax you stop, you enjoy the moment, without being caught unprepared by what is usually called the refractory period and which leads to post-coitus sleepiness. Then? You might be overwhelmed by hours of welfare. Because also your soul - of course, in addition to your body - has found satisfaction in what happens between the sheets.

The secret is that there is nothing that needs to be done to get to the Valley orgasm. The only difficulty is that you don't have to do anything. Usually when you make love you are tense, often the face is serious, sometimes even dramatic. We are worried, we want to make a good impression and we don't know how it will end. Here, the difficulty is just this: you don't have to worry about how it ends, nor that your penis is erect.

It is enough for me to stay inside the partner. It is not even necessary to move: simple intimate contact is sufficient. One must be with the muscles of the whole body abandoned, man must not attempt to sustain an erection in any way; must not contract the pelvic muscles. Instead the woman, if she wants, can move the vaginal muscles. One thing that can happen is that the woman, despite not reaching orgasm, feels satisfied.

The trigger mechanism is basically physiological in nature and goes hand in hand with a pre-existing psychological relaxation situation. If the position is held for at least thirty-five minutes, a physical reaction occurs, causing the brain waves of both lovers to adjust to a general level and be very calm. In other words, physiological reactions, physical changes that occur in our body. Therefore, one must not make the mistake of considering the experience of tantra as something mystical, ideal, mental.

When someone is actively doing something and is tense, the brain works in short and fast wave rhythms. In this state, the body's ability to feel pleasant sensations is bad because the mind requires a lot of energy to dry the body and vital organs. When you relax the rhythm of the brain's work, it slows down and the waves that characterize it continue to elongate.

In this state, the energies consumed by the mind are very few and the organism can use all the available forces to optimize itself and cure any malfunctions. In the case of a couple who experiences the experience of tantric sex (but this can be true for any situation in which they share a relaxing situation and sensations) brain waves not only slow down but tune in to the same "length D 'wave". In short, you have to give yourself and your body time to tune in to your partner.

Especially for the sexual encounter between two partners finding oneself in a situation of unity in which there is no anxiety to obtain a result, and therefore relaxing, together with the wet contact that occurs between the genital organs and the bodily approach allows maximum contact, makes the establishment of this unity feel stronger. And this is precisely what allows the ecstasy.

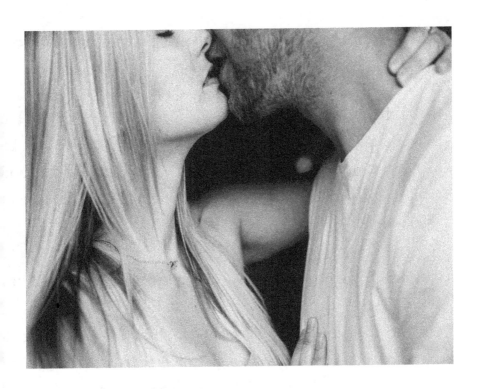

Chapter 15. Sexual health: preserve an active and satisfying sex life

If you don't neglect your sexual well-being, your quality of life will improve. This is an important aspect and should not be underestimated because it affects physical, mental and emotional health. An active sex life is actually an indicator of good health.

Physical, mental and social conditions related to sexuality

This requires positive commitment and respect for sexuality and sexual relations as well as the opportunity to have a pleasant and safe sexual experience without coercion, discrimination and violence. This is what the World Health Organization defines sexual well-being.

At the biological level, sexual energy interferes with the brain's oxygen supply, hormonal balance, respiration and stress reduction, and muscle tension. In fact, recent research shows that sex with certain patterns can increase life expectancy. This is due to hormonal effects such as DHEA, a hormone which, in addition to stimulating sexual function, also controls the production of myelin, an important substance to protect and function of the nervous system.

However, on a psychological level, a good sexual health surely increases self-confidence and intimacy. In fact, sex has the ability to eliminate anxiety and anxiety and increase relaxation and well-being. This is mainly caused by endorphins, protein hormones that act as neurotransmitters and affect mood and happiness, and help fight depression.

The importance of healthy sexual habits

However, to be able to enjoy all the beneficial effects, it is necessary to maintain healthy sexual habits. In fact, sexual contact is not only based on penetration techniques, which are not the most important or even the purpose of the relationship itself. You don't even have to have too much hope. Instead, it is necessary to start from a state of mental relaxation and enjoy the sensations that arise during sexual intercourse. Satisfaction, love, desire, pleasure and love help create healthy and rewarding life experiences and experience our sexuality more intensely. Suppressing or ignoring a person's sexual health means being unable to enjoy, which limits one's desires and needs.

Sports useful for improving sexual performance

What is the relationship between sports and sex? Running, fitness, and yoga are disciplines that can help couples have sex. Sports and sex are very solid units that can influence each other.

Indeed, healthy exercise not only helps couples physically face physical actions, but above all triggers various chemical reactions that make the body more vulnerable to sex. But which sports improve sexual performance for her and him? We find running, fitness and yoga!

You don't have to train for a marathon, but running from time to time is definitely one of the physical exercises that helps improve sexual performance. First of all, it helps to tighten your body and you know that if you feel comfortable with your body, you tend to be more confident with your partner. In addition, running is an aerobic discipline that increases endurance by exercising the heart.

Not everyone may like running, for physical reasons, someone may be looking for a gentler exercise for their body. In this case, cycling or swimming are two excellent alternatives to train your body in a harmonious way both from a muscular point of view, and going to look for a type of training aimed at increasing heart beats. The link between these two sports and sexual performance is very interesting as cycling and swimming are disciplines that unite partners also empathetically. The bike is an extremely pleasant sport to do with your loved one as it is possible to organize beautiful couple outings in suggestive places. After a swim, however, the ideal is to jump into the hot tub and relax with your loved one.

Fitness is also a core discipline in the combination of sports and sexual performance. Special whole body training units for muscle training lead to increased desire and vitality that is stronger during sexual intercourse, especially in men. In addition, energetic and reinforced physics significantly improves performance. Anyone who believes that yoga is a woman's sport must change his mind. Actually, yoga not only makes the body smoother and more flexible, but for disciplined people it carves the upper body, strengthens the legs and defines the back. However, this helps the couple find harmony and inner well-being.

The libido foods
Food and sex have several points in common:

- They represent intense and fulfilling pleasures, natural and generally available to everyone;
- They are linked by the symbolic aspect of sociality: you eat, enjoy and have sex with other people. In fact, when there was no sharing, both behaviors would not be well viewed;

- They are linked to the concept of self-control;
- They are fundamental for survival and evolution;
- They are co-localized anatomically and biochemically.

Men and women are always looking for foods that stimulate sexual desire. Things are changed many times over the centuries. From Castore Durante, a 16th-century italian doctor that recommended singing, while Catherine de Medici, Queen o. France, focused on thorns, onions, beans, zucchini, celery onions, mushrooms, and artichokes made in grapes.

Spices like cinnamon, red pepper and black pepper, but spices like ginger always have a good reputation in sexual field. Maybe there is a background truth because they stimulate blood circulation. Another way to focus is on foods that are male (asparagus) or female (seafood). But as always, it depends on the imagination to get ready! One thing is certain: if you tickle the palate with delicious food, the endorphin content increases. The most important thing is to try what you have in front of you, or to have fun, why not that we are the main dish, which allows the couple to use himself as a table or main dish, provided he follows the instincts of the couple and observes the couple and this personal taste.

Feed and reproduction are two important functions for the conservation of the human species and are therefore valued by nature with maximum pleasure. So food and sex are always connected in the culture of every nation and in every historical era.

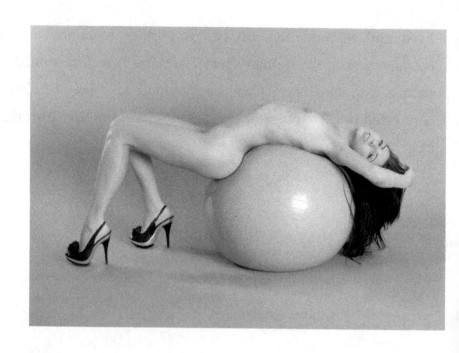

Conclusion

There are many advantages to tantra, because this discipline works at all levels of the individual. The purpose of teaching is not only to gain more knowledge, but also to become more aware of ourselves and the behaviors we use. From a sexual standpoint, we become more aware of ourselves and our preferences and significantly increase through the teachings we learn, the way we love. We can turn sexuality into a very profound spiritual experience and achieve ultimate pleasure by trying to achieve a deep tantric ecstasy.

From the point of view of love and partner, we can better understand the people we love and understand the uniqueness and beauty of the aspects of men and women. Let's rediscover what is surviving partner and think about the nature of true love, which is very altruistic. We learn to build deeper, more harmonious and fulfilling relationships with loved ones and use partners as powerful tools for evolution and transformation.

But the benefits aren't just that; Indeed, because you will practice yoga exercises, meditation techniques, tantric pairing techniques, mindfulness exercises and mantras. You will keep benefit emotionally from physical plans (having a stronger and healthier bodies), mental plans (more relaxed and harmonious thoughts - you will be balanced and focused) and spiritual.

Through the techniques you have learned in this book, partners can have the most out-of-body experience on a larger scale. This is possible by increasing the senses. Therefore, the ritual performed in the act of love is the best moment where the individual reaches the peak of pleasure, not only his own pleasure, but also the pleasure of others.

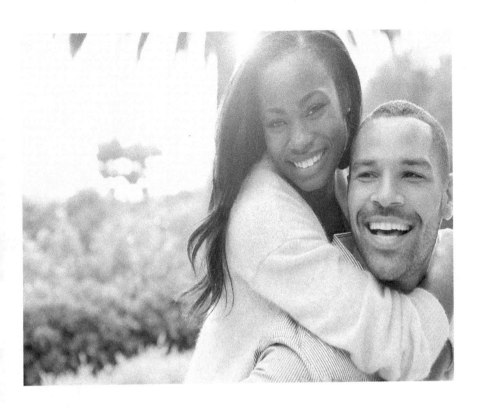

CPSIA information can be obtained
at www.ICGtesting.com
Printed in the USA
LVHW081032180121
676360LV00040B/338